Essential Oils

Bible for Beginners

More Than 250 Recipes for Anti-aging, Weight loss, Skin, Hair and Health Care

Copyright © 2016

by Andrew Costei

Copyright notice

No part of this book may be reproduced or transmitted in any form or by any means, electronic or mechanical, including photocopying, recording or by any information storage and retrieval system, without written permission from the author.

General Disclaimers

This book contains information that is intended to help the readers be better informed consumers of health care. It is presented as general advice on health care and is not intended to be a substitute for the medical advice of a licensed physician. The reader should consult with their doctor in any matters relating to his/her health.

Although the author and publisher have made every effort to ensure that the information in this book was correct at press time, the author and publisher do not assume and hereby disclaim any liability to any party for any loss, damage, or disruption caused by errors or omissions, whether such errors or omissions result from negligence, accident, or any other cause.

Contents

Essential oils. What they are? 15

    Main components 15

    The physiological significance of essential oils. 15

    The use of essential oils 16

    Priority properties include the following effects. 16

    A bit of theory about the essential and base oils..17

    How base oils action on the skin?..17

    KEY FEATURES OF BASE OILS..17

    Security measures. 17

    The main base oils..18

    Rules of Use..18

    Rules of Dilution 20

Baths with essential oils. How to take baths, recipes 22

    The use of essential oils 22

    How to take a bath with essential oils 22

Dill Oil. Useful properties and applications of dill oil..25

    The composition and obtaining of the essential oil from dill. 25

    Action and uses of dill oil 25

    Dill oil for weight correction...26

    Contraindications for dill oil...27

Marigold oil: Properties and applications for hair and face.......................................27

    Application of calendula oil...28

    Calendula oil for the face 28

    Calendula oil for hair..29

Oils for protection from the sun and tanning (against UV-radiation).UV-protective properties of oils...........30

    What oil protect skin from the sun and tanning? 31

    How to use the oil to protect from the sun and tanning? 31

    Essential oils for tanning. 31

    Essential oils that are harmful during tanning. 32

    Essential oils to get a good tan...33

    Essential oils to protect against UV...33

    The use of essential oils for sunburn. 33

Castor oil. Properties and application of castor oil. 34

    Properties of castor oil. 35

    Application of castor oil. 35

    Laxative properties of castor oil. 36

    Treatment with castor oil. 36

    The use of castor oil for the skin. 36

    Castor oil in mixtures. 37

Thyme oil. Treatment and use of essential oil of thyme in cosmetology. 37

    The essential oil of thyme 38

    Oil from thyme for Treatment 39

    The use of thyme oil in cosmetics. 40

Oil of lemon balm. Properties and application of essential oil of lemon balm 40

    Properties of lemon balm oil. 41

    Application of lemon balm oil. 41

    Oil of lemon balm in dermatology 42

    Oil of lemon balm for lips 42

    Oil of lemon balm for the skin 42

    Oil of lemon balm for hair 43

    Baths with lemon balm oil. 43

Cocoa butter: composition and properties of the treatment. 44

    Cacao oil 44

    Cocoa butter treatment 45

    Cocoa butter in the home cosmetics 46

Celandine oil: composition, useful properties. The use and treatment of essential oil of celandine. 47

    The composition of the oil of celandine. 48

    Useful properties of celandine 48

    The use of celandine oil. 49

Essential oil from Frankincense: application, useful properties and composition. 50

    The composition of essential oils of frankincense 50

    Use of frankincense fragrance 51

    The use of essential oil of frankincense 51

The essential oil of myrrh. The composition, properties and applications of myrrh oil. 52

    The properties of essential oil of myrrh 53

    The use of myrrh oil 54

Thistle oil. Application properties and contraindications for thistle oil..55

  The use of thistle oil 55

  Thistle oil properties 56

  Thistle oil in cosmetics 57

Rosehip oil: structure, properties, application, treatment. Rosehip oil in cosmetology: for the face, décolleté, hair and stretch marks. 57

  Rosehip oil: Composition 58

  Rosehip oil: Properties, use and treatment 58

  Rosehip oil in cosmetology: For the face, neck and the hair 59

  Oil of rose hips as a remedy for stretch marks 59

Essential oils for sleeping (insomnia). Massage, oil burner and internal use of essential oils to sleep............60

  Essential oils for sleep..60

  Massage with essential oils for sleep..61

  Aroma with essential oils for insomnia 61

  Internal use of essential oils for sleep..62

  Baths with essential oils for sleep 62

  Contraindications to the use of essential oils for a dream 62

Essential oil of nutmeg: composition and properties. Muscat oil in cosmetics, cooking and aromatherapy. .63

  Composition and healing properties of nutmeg oil 63

  Muscat oil in case of problems with digestion...64

  Muscat oil in cooking 64

  Muscat oil in cosmetics 65

  Nutmeg oil in aromatherapy...65

Apricot kernel oil: structure, properties and applications. Apricot kernel oil in cosmetics for the face, hair and nails. 66

  The composition of apricot kernel oil 66

  Apricot kernel oil: properties, application, treatment..66

  Apricot kernel oil in cosmetics.For hair, nails and skin 67

  Recipes with apricot kernel oil 67

Peach oil: chemical composition and properties of peach oil. The use of peach oil. Mask with peach oil for the skin and eyelashes. 69

  The chemical composition of peach oil...69

  The properties of peach butter...69

  Contraindications for peach oil 70

  Mask with peach butter to the face and body..70

Lotion with peach butter..71

Mask with peach butter to the hair 71

Essential oil of citronella: composition and properties of citronella oil. Use of citronella oil. 71

Essential oil of citronella: composition 72

Properties and application of essential oils of citronella 72

Contraindications for citronella oil...73

Influence of citronella oil on the psycho-emotional state 73

Essential oil of citronella: methods of application 73

Chamomile essential oil: composition, useful properties and applications of chamomile oil. Chamomile oil for hair use, cosmetics, skin and nails. 74

The composition of the essential oil of chamomile 74

Chamomile essential oil: useful properties, application 75

Contraindications 75

The use of chamomile essential oil in cosmetics, for hair, skin and nails.......................................76

Stone oil: chemical composition, the use and contraindications. stone oil treatment. Crack stone oil. 76

The chemical composition of the stone oil 77

Contraindications to the use of stone oil..77

Stone oil treatment: application 77

Cure from stone oil...78

Application for the treatment of stone oil..78

Anise oil: composition. Useful properties and treatment with essential oil of anise. The use of anise oil in cosmetics for the face, body and hair. 80

Anise oil: composition 80

Essential oil of anise: useful properties, treatment 80

Mixture for massage with anise oil for skin tightening 81

Mango butter: composition, properties, application, and treatment. Essential oil of mango in cosmetics for the face, body and hair. 82

Mango oil: composition 83

Mango butter: properties, use and treatment 83

Oil from Mango for hair 84

Mango butter for the face and body..84

Neroli: properties and composition. Contraindications and warnings for the use of essential oil of neroli. Neroli for skin use. 85

Types of neroli oil...85

The properties and composition of the essential oil of neroli 85

The composition of essential oil of Neroli 86

Contraindications and warnings for the use of neroli...86

Neroli oil for skin 86

Application of neroli oil 87

Geranium oil: composition, properties and treatment with geranium oil. Geranium essential oils in cosmetics, for skin, face and hair. 88

Essential oil of geranium: composition and properties 88

Essential oil of geranium at home...89

Treatment with essential oil of geranium: folk recipes 89

Essential oil of geranium in cosmetology: geranium oil for the skin, face and hair 90

Essential oil of geranium: contraindications 90

St. John's Wort Oil: Composition and healing properties. St. John's wort oil in cosmetics. Indications and contraindications for the use of essential oil from St. John's wort..90

The composition and useful properties of St. John's wort 91

Preparation St. John's Wort oil: the first recipe..91

The use of St. John's wort oil...91

Preparation of St. John's Wort oil: second recipe...91

The use of St. John's wort oil...91

St. John's wort oil in cosmetics 92

The therapeutic effect of St. John's wort oil 92

Contraindications 93

Avocado oil: structure and advantageous properties. Uses of avocado oil. Avocado oil in hair cosmetics, eyelashes, face and hands...93

Avocado oil: structure and advantageous properties..93

The use of avocado oil..94

Avocado oil in cosmetics for hair, eyelashes, face and hands 94

Recipes for avocado oil in cosmetics...95

Linseed oil: healing and medicinal properties, treatment. Linseed oil in cosmetics, for the face, body and hair. 96

The healing properties of flaxseed oil 96

Medicinal properties of linseed oil..96

The useful linseed oil...96

With what is useful to use linseed oil 97

The fatty acids in linseed oil 97

Treatment with linseed oil: folk recipes..97

Linseed oil in cosmetics for face and body 99

Linseed oil for hands 99

Linseed oil for face and body skin...99

Linseed oil for hair..99

Mustard oil: structure, benefits, features, treatment, and contraindications. The use of mustard oil in cosmetics for the face and hair. 100

Mustard oil: composition, properties and use...100

Vitamins in mustard oil 101

Mustard oil: indications and treatment with mustard oil...102

Contraindications for mustard oil 102

Mustard oil: uses in cosmetics for the face and hair 102

Hazelnut oil: composition, properties. Hazelnut oil in cosmetics and cooking: recipes...................103

The composition of the hazelnut oil 103

Energy value of hazelnut oil 103

The properties of hazelnut oil 104

Traditional recipes with hazelnut oil...105

Oil hazelnut in cooking..106

Cinnamon oil: composition, properties and use. Use and treatment with cinnamon oil. The essential oil of cinnamon in cosmetology and cooking...106

Cinnamon Essential Oil: composition..106

Features and benefits of essential oil of cinnamon 107

The use and treatment with essential oil of cinnamon 107

The essential oil of cinnamon in cosmetology 108

The essential oil of cinnamon in cooking 108

Sandalwood essential oil: structure, benefits, use and treatment with sandalwood oil. Sandalwood oil in cosmetics, for the face, hands, nails and hair..109

Essential oil of sandalwood: composition...109

Sandalwood oil: the use, application and treatment. Properties of sandalwood oil 109

Sandalwood oil in cosmetics for the face, hands, hair and nails 110

Essential oil of pine: the benefits, indications, the use and treatment with pine oil. Pine oil in cosmetics for the face, hands and hair...111

Essential oil of pine: the use, treatment and indications...111

Contraindications for pine oil...112

Essential oil of pine: application...112

Oil in cosmetics for the face, hands and hair..113

Shea butter: properties and composition. The use of shea butter in cosmetics and at home: creams and masks..114

The composition of shea butter...114

Properties and treatment with shea butter...114

The use of shea butter in cosmetics..115

Creams based on shea butter 116

Masks based on shea butter 116

Shea oil for Hair...117

Contraindications for shea butter 117

Essential oil of fennel: the use, application, properties and treatment. Fennel oil in hair cosmetics, facial skin, body and hands...117

Fennel oil: the use and application 118

Properties of fennel oil..118

Fennel Oil for Treatment..118

Contraindications to the use of fennel oil...119

Essential oil of fir: composition and properties. The use and treatment with fir oil. 120

Essential oil of fir: composition and properties 120

The use and treatment wtih pine oil...121

Fir oil against toothache...121

Baths with essential oils of fir 122

Contraindications for fir essential oil 122

Essential oil of bergamot: properties, use and contraindications. Essential oil of bergamot in cosmetology. 122

The properties of essential oil of bergamot...123

The use of essential oil of bergamot..123

Essential oil of bergamot in cosmetology 123

Bergamot oil for the body 124

Treatment with oil of bergamot..124

The essential oil of ginger: the use, structure, properties and applications. Ginger oil in skin and hair cosmetics...124

The use of ginger oil...125

The use and composition of essential oil of ginger..125

The properties of essential oil of ginger 125

The essential oil of ginger in cosmetology 126

How to prepare ginger oil at home 126

9

Walnut oil: structure, properties, application, and treatment. Walnut oil in cosmetics for skin and hair, tanning and slimming. 127

Walnut oil: structure and properties 127

The use of walnut oil 127

Treatment with walnut oil...127

Walnut oil in cosmetics for skin and hair 128

Walnut oil for tanning 129

Walnut oil for weight loss 129

Essential oil of cypress: properties, use, indications and contraindications. Cypress oil in cosmetics for skin, hair, hands and nails. 129

Properties of cypress oil..129

Benefits and indications for cypress oil 130

Cypress oil for the skin 130

Cypress oil for hair...130

Contraindications for cypress oil...131

Recipes with cypress oil 131

Cedar oil: useful properties, treatment, use. Cedar oil in cosmetics, for face, hands, nails and hair. 132

Useful properties of cedar oil..132

Treatment with cedar oil...133

The use of cedar oil 133

Essential oil of mandarin: composition and properties. The use and treatment with mandarin oil. Essential oil of tangerine in cosmetology..134

The composition of essential oils of mandarin 134

Properties of mandarin oil 134

The use of essential oils of mandarin..135

Essential oil of tangerine in cosmetology 136

Sea buckthorn oil: A useful composition, the use and treatment with sea buckthorn oil. Recipes with sea buckthorn. 136

A useful composition of sea buckthorn oil...137

Treatment with sea buckthorn oil. Recipes with Sea Buckthorn 137

Face masks with sea buckthorn oil 139

How to cook sea buckthorn oil...139

Sage essential oil: structure, properties, application to hair, skin, hands and nails. Treatment with oil of sage. 140

The composition of the essential oil of sage...140

Treatment with sage oil 141

Essential oil of sage for hair 141

Sage oil for the skin 141

Sage oil for hands and nails 142

Peppermint essential oil: the use, composition and properties. The use of essential oil of mint: recipes from peppermint oil...142

The composition of the essential oil of peppermint 143

The use of essential oil of mint: recipes from peppermint oil 143

Contraindications for peppermint oil...144

Grape seed oil: Structure, properties and applications. Grape seed oil for face and body...........................145

The use of grape seed oil 145

The composition of grape seed oil 146

The cosmetic use of grape seed oil, as a separate ingredient, or as a supplement in the various cosmetic preparations..146

Grape seed oil for face and body 146

Wheat germ oil: properties and benefits. Wheat germ oil for face, hair (mask) and stretch marks.............147

Properties and benefits of wheat germ oil 147

The use of wheat germ oil in cosmetics 148

Wheat germ oil for the face 149

Wheat germ oil for hair..149

Prevention and treatment of diseases with wheat germ oil..150

Contraindications to the use of wheat oil..150

The conditions of storage of wheat germ oil 150

Grapefruit essential oil: composition and use. Grapefruit oil in cosmetology and facial hair. Indications and contraindications of grapefruit oil. 150

The composition and the use of essential oil of grapefruit 151

Grapefruit essential oil in cosmetics 151

The essential oil of grapefruit - help in everyday life...152

Contraindications grapefruit oil 152

Lavender essential oil: structure, benefits, treatment with lavender oil. Lavender essential oil in cosmetology: for hands, nails, skin and hair 152

The composition of the essential oil of lavender..153

Properties and healing action of the essential oil of lavender 153

The use of lavender oil for medicinal purposes 154

The use of lavender oil in cosmetics 154

Lavender essential oil for skin, hair, hands, nails...155

11

Lemon essential oil: structure, benefits, treatment of lemon oil. The use of essential oil of lemon in cosmetics for skin, hair and nails. 155

The composition and preparation of essential oil of lemon 156

Properties of essential oil of lemon 156

The action and the application of recipes essential oil of lemon 157

The use of lemon essential oil in cosmetics 158

Lemon essential oil for the skin 158

Lemon oil for hair 158

Rose essential oil: the use and composition. Useful properties of rose oil in medicine and cosmetology. Homemade recipes and treatment with essential oil of rose...159

Raw materials for essential oil rose 159

The composition of essential rose oil...159

The use of essential oil of roses in medicine and cosmetology 160

Homemade recipes for the use of essential oil of rose 160

Clove essential oil: composition, useful properties and applications. Essential oil of clove for hair and skin: recipes. 161

The composition of the clove essential oil...161

Useful properties and applications of clove essential oil..162

Essential oil of cloves for hair: recipes 162

Clove essential oil for skin: recipes 163

Other recipes with essential oil of clove 163

Eucalyptus essential oil: structure, properties and application of recipes. Eucalyptus essential for the skin, nails and hair oil. 164

The composition of the essential oil of eucalyptus. Production of eucalyptus oil 164

The properties of essential oil of eucalyptus 164

The use of eucalyptus oil...164

Use of eucalyptus oil 165

Treatment with essential oil of eucalyptus..165

Recipes with essential oil of eucalyptus...165

The use of essential oil of eucalyptus in cosmetology...166

Eucalyptus essential oils for the skin, hands, nails and hair 166

Tea tree essential oil: composition and therapeutic properties Directions for use and treatment with essential tea tree oil..167

The composition of the essential oil of tea tree 167

Medicinal properties of tea tree essential oil 167

The use of essential oil of tea tree 168

Methods of application of tea tree oil. Tea Tree Oil Treatment 169

Essential oil of orange: the use, action and therapeutic properties. Essential oil of orange for skin and cellulite. 170

The history of essential oil of orange 170

The use of essential oil of orange 171

Orange oil for skin, cellulite 171

The healing properties of essential oils of orange 171

Emotional effect of essential oil of orange 172

Essential oil of orange: precautions 172

Dosage of essential oil of orange 172

Essential oil of Jojoba: the use, benefits and properties. Essential oil of Jojoba for skin and hair. Recipes with jojoba oil. 173

Jojoba oil - the arguments "for" 173

Jojoba oil for skin care 173

Composition of jojoba oil 173

Jojoba Oil Properties 174

The action of jojoba oil 174

Jojoba oil for hair 174

Jojoba oil at home. Recipes with jojoba oil 175

Essential oil of ylang-ylang: an aphrodisiac and use in cosmetology. Medicinal properties and application of essential oil from ylang-ylang. 176

Essential oil of ylang-ylang - aphrodisiac 176

Essential oil of ylang-ylang in cosmetology 176

Cure properties of essential oil of ylang-ylang 177

Essential oil of ylang-ylang and the human psyche 177

Essential oil of ylang-ylang: impact on sexuality 177

Terms of use of the essential oil from ylang-ylang 178

The essential oil of rosemary. Properties, application, contraindications and treatment with essential oil of rosemary. Hair masks with rosemary 178

The properties of essential oil of rosemary 178

The use and treatment with essential oil of rosemary 179

Rosemary essential oil in cosmetics 180

Indications of rosemary essential oil 180

Contraindications for the use of essential oil of rosemary 180

Rosemary essential oil for hair: mask with rosemary 181

Patchouli essential oil. Production, use and properties of essential oil of patchouli. Patchouli essential oils for the face: masks, steam baths. 181

Preparation of essential oil of patchouli 182

The use of essential oil of patchouli 182

Properties of patchouli essential oil 182

Methods of application of essential oil of patchouli..183

Patchouli essential oils for the face: for mask, steam baths...184

Essential oils. What they are?

Essential oil (oil) - volatile, with a strong characteristic odor and flavor, oil-like (oily), insoluble in water, basically colorless or weakly colored liquid. Unlike real fats they do not leave greasy stains on paper because evaporate (volatilize), even at room temperature. Essential oils are formed only in plants, but they have extremely strong physiological and pharmacological properties. In pure form, they are produced by steam distillation, absorbed by fats, somewhere squeezed under pressure, or extracted with liquid carbon dioxide and other solvents. In phytotherapy (aromatherapy) they are used not only in purified form, such as for inhalation, but in tinctures (essences) which are to make from alcohol, terpenes from them are insoluble in water, or steams. Most essential oils are readily soluble by alcohol (solubility of essential oils in an alcohol strongly depends on its strength), gasoline, ether lipids and fatty oils, waxes and other lipophilic substances, and such forms are widely used in perfumery (Perfume and cosmetic industry). Essential oils are also used in the food industry - as herbs and spices.

Essential oils are distinguished and referred to as the plants from which they are derived: peppermint, lavender, pink and others. Each of them is a mixture of several (often more) of certain chemical compounds - terpenes and their derivatives (terpenoids). Terpenes - hydrocarbons, characterized by the fact that many molecules have unsaturated carbon bonds that cause high chemical activity of these substances.

Main components

The composition of essential oils includes terpenes, terpenoids, aromatics, saturated and unsaturated hydrocarbons, aldehydes, organic acids and alcohols, esters and heterocyclic compounds, amines, phenols, organic sulfides, oxides and others.

The choice of essential oils depends on the quality indicators of the scope of application, and is determined by their naturalness, perfume, pharmacological and taste- aromatic properties.

Composition of essential oils depends on the plant species, it chemotype, weather conditions in the year of collection, storage conditions of the raw material, the method of extraction of essential oils, and often the duration and storage conditions

The physiological significance of essential oils.

Essential oils are widely distributed in the plant world, and their role is very great. The most important physiological functions include the following:

1. Essential oils are the active metabolites of metabolic processes occurring in the plant body. In favor of this judgment shows high reactivity terpenoid and aromatic compounds, which are the main components of the essential oils.

2. Essential oils upon evaporation envelop the plant in a kind of "cushion", reducing air heat transfer, which promotes prevention of plants from excessive heat during the day and at night hypothermia, as well as the regulation of transpiration.

3. Smells of plants used to attract pollinators-insects, which helps pollinate the flowers.

4. Essential oils can prevent infection by pathogenic fungi and bacteria, and also protect the plants from being eaten by animals.

The use of essential oils
1. food flavorings;
2. medicines, pharmaceuticals;
3. components of perfumes and toilet preparations (cosmetology);
4. aromatherapy;
5. and other like solvents.

Priority properties include the following effects.
1. The antimicrobial (antibacterial, antiseptic) properties (the leaves of eucalyptus, poplar buds, clove oil, pine oil, and others).
2. The anti-inflammatory properties (camphor, chamomile flowers, yarrow, elecampane rhizomes and others).
3. Antispasmodic activity (peppermint leaves, chamomile flowers, coriander, dill, and others).
4. Expectorant (shoots of wild rosemary, fennel and anise fruits, roots of elecampane, thyme, oregano grass, and others).
5. Sedation (rhizomes of valerian, lemon balm herb, lavender flowers, and others).
6. Diuretic properties (buds and leaves of birch, juniper fruit, and others).
7. Regenerating action (hamazulen flowers, chamomile, and others).

A bit of theory about the essential and base oils

All oils that we can apply in our masks, body wraps can be divided into 2 types: essential and vegetable (basic) oil. All essential oils are sold in dark glass small (5-10 ml) jars. Base oils are sold in dark glass (plastic) jars of 50 ml or more. In turn, the base oils can be liquid or solid (shea butter (Karite)), coconut oil, cocoa butter, mango butter - it is better not to buy refined).

All essential oils must be mixed with the base oil. The exception is tea tree oil and lavender - they can be used without the base oils.

Essential oils are selected by the smell - *if you do not like the smell of oil, it will not work with you.*

How base oils action on the skin?

Today, the base oil, added to cosmetics, not only serve as bases, but also as biologically active components, which not only provide other oils penetration into the skin, but do affect physiological processes in the skin. Particularly valuable in this respect, are oils containing essential fatty acid: linoleic, alpha-linolenic and gamma linolenic (Omega 3 and Omega 6).

For normal skin, these acids operation, must be ingested in the correct ratio, the range of 4:1-1:1. With a lack of these acids, the skin starts to peel off, it becomes dry and irritated.

The base oil composition can also contain valuable components such as carotenoids, phytosterols, squalene, tocopherol.

KEY FEATURES OF BASE OILS

1) Formation of the epidermal barrier (fats are needed for the formation of the lipid layers of the corneum stratum);

2) participation in the metabolism of biologically active molecules;

3) Increasing the permeability of the corneum stratum for other active ingredients.

Security measures.

Keep in mind that essential oils have a very powerful effect, and require careful handling. In particular, the essential oils can not be applied to the skin in pure form - it must first be diluted with base oil. After contact with skin, the oil must to be cleaned immediately. Admission of essential oil inside can cause severe poisoning. Essential oils should be stored out of the reach of children and animals. It is necessary to protect eyes from getting in them the essential oils. In the case of contact with eyes or mucous, rinse immediately with plenty of water and seek medical advice.

Essential oils should be purchased only from proven and reliable sources, before applying make sure, in accordance with the content label, follow the enclosed instructions.

The main base oils
1. Wheat germ oil;
2. Jojoba oil;
3. Granet seed oil;
4. Olive oil;
5. Coconut oil;
6. Oil of aloe vera;
7. Avocado oil;
8. Castor oil;
9. Grape seed oil;
10. Cranberry;
11. Apricot kernel oil;
12. Linseed oil;
13. Almond oil;
14. Shi oil

The most soft oils: *almond oil, jojoba oil, macadamia oil.*

Rules of Use
1. Buy from companies that provide directions for use on the label.
2. Carrier oils can be used to dilute your essential oils. Some are coconut, olive, grapeseed, Vitamin E oil, and some vegetable oils. This ensures that when the oils are applied to your skin they will be smooth and comfortable. The essential oils are not diluted with carrier oils. The full benefit is there and if you want them diluted with carrier oils, you can do it as you want it.
3. Do not use oils with petroleum products that can be mineral oil, petroleum jelly baby oil, vegetable shortening, butter, or margarine. These are not carrier oils.

4. Before using oils on your skin do a patch test in a small area on your arm. Some oils for example clove, cinnamon, lemongrass, thyme, oregano, and peppermint can have a cool or hot sensation that people do not like or are sensitive to.

5. For a patch test put one or two drops of the oils on your lower arm. Wait a few hours to see if there is any effect that should appear within 5 to 10 minutes. If you feel cool, hot or have a rash, use a carrier oil to alleviate this condition the next time you use the oil.

6. When you have any discomfort on your skin, discontinue using the oil. Carrier oils mixed with the essential oil should work to alleviate this problem.

7. If you get essential oils in your eye, see your ophthalmologist (eye doctor) immediately.

8. Never use water to flush the eyes and skin sensitivities. Water makes it worse.

9. Do not use essential oils at the ears, eyes, mucous membranes around lips and nose, or the genital area.

10. Essential oils at sensitive areas can be diluted with 5 to 10 drops of carrier oil. Some essential oil companies offer carrier oils.

11. If you are a newbie to essential oils, start out slowly with a few drops and increase the amount over time.

12. If you are pregnant or nursing, check with your healthcare provider, pharmacist, or aromatherapist before using essential oils.

13. Babies and youngsters can use some essential oils and they should be diluted with carrier oils. Rub baby's feet and be sure you purchase oils made specifically for children to be safe.

14. Some citrus oils have components that can react to ultraviolet (UV) rays from the sun. This photosensitivity might cause a reaction for you. Be sure to read the labels where UV rays are indicated for the product (photosensitivity) and stay out of the sun.

15. If you take prescription medicines, be sure to check with an aromatherapist, a pharmacist, or healthcare provider for contraindications. Some drugs can interact with essential oils.

Rules of Dilution

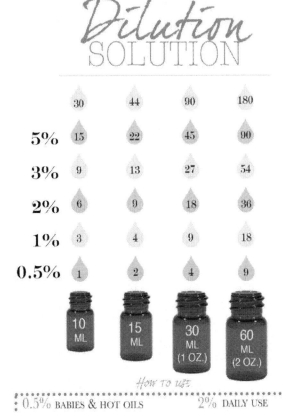

Dilution
SOLUTION

	30	44	90	180
5%	15	22	45	90
3%	9	13	27	54
2%	6	9	18	36
1%	3	4	9	18
0.5%	1	2	4	9
	10 ML	15 ML	30 ML (1 OZ.)	60 ML (2 OZ.)

How to use

0.5% BABIES & HOT OILS   2% DAILY USE

1% KIDS, ELDERLY, SENSITIVE   5-10% SHORT TERM

Neat = Straight, undiluted
Dilution usually NOT required; suitable for all but the most sensitive skin. Safe for children over 2 years old.

50-50 = Dilute 50-50
Dilution recommended at 50-50 (1 part essential oils to 1 part V-6 Vegetable Oil Complex) for topical and internal use, especially when used on sensitive areas – face, neck, genital area, underarms, etc. Keep out of reach of children.

20-80 = Dilute 20-80
Always dilute 20-80 (1 part essential oils to 4 parts V-6 Vegetable Oil Complex) before applying to the skin or taking internally. Keep out of reach of children.

PH = Photosensitising
Avoid using on skin exposed to direct sunlight or UV rays (i.e. sunlamps, tanning beds, etc.)

Balsam Fir (Idaho)	50-50	Galbanum	Neat	Patchouli	Neat
Basil	50-50	Geranium	50-50	Peppermint	50-50
Bergamot	50-50 PH	Ginger	50-50	Petitgrain	Neat
Black Pepper	50-50	Goldenrod	50-50	Pine	50-50
Cassia	20-80	Grapefruit	50-50 PH	Ravensara	50-50
Cedarwood	Neat	Helichrysum	50-50	Roman Chamomile	Neat
Cinnamon Bark	20-80	Hyssop	20-80	Rose	Neat
Cistus	Neat	Jasmine	Neat	Rosemary	50-50
Clary Sage	50-50	Juniper	50-50	Rosewood	Neat
Clove	20-80	Laurus nobilis or Bay Laurel	50-50	Sacred Frankincense	50-50
Copaiba	Neat	Lavender	Neat	Sage	50-50
Coriander	50-50	Ledum	Neat	Sandalwood	Neat
Cypress	50-50	Lemon	50-50 PH	Spearmint	50-50
Dill	50-50	Lemongrass	20-80	Spikenard	Neat
Dorado Azul	50-50	Marjoram	50-50	Spruce	50-50
Douglas Fir	50-50	Melaleuca (M. alternifolia)	50-50	Tangerine	50-50 PH
Elemi	Neat	Melissa	Neat	Tarragon	50-50
Eucalyptus Blue (E bicostata)	50-50	Mountain Savory	50-50	Thyme	20-80
Eucalyptus (E citriodora)	50-50	Myrrh	Neat	Tsuga	50-50
Eucalyptus (E dives)	50-50	Myrtle	50-50	Valerian	Neat
Eucalyptus (E globulus)	50-50	Nutmeg	50-50	Vetiver	Neat
Eucalyptus (E polybractea)	50-50	Ocotea	20-80	Western Red Cedar	50-50
Eucalyptus (E radiata)	50-50	Orange	50-50 PH	White Fir	50-50
Fennel	Neat	Oregano	20-80	Wintergreen	50-50
Frankincense	50-50	Palo Santo	50-50	Ylang Ylang	Neat

Tab.1.Dilution of essential oils

Baths with essential oils. How to take baths, recipes

Every day, women have to overcome many difficulties, remodel a huge pile of cases. And often in the evening we can not stop all the running, running somewhere. From such a life rhythm sleep deteriorates, there is a constant feeling of fatigue, lethargy and low mood. How to avoid these unpleasant phenomena? Very simple. Stop and finally take the time his beloved. One of the easiest ways - a scented bath with essential oils. You do not need to prepare anything in advance, do not need to spend a lot of time for the procedure. And the effect of such baths will surpass all expectations. After all, they help not only to relax, but also have a beauty and even healing effect.

Aromatic bath was used since ancient times - not so much for leisure as for treatment. After all, our ancestors knew better than us what is hidden in the healing power of herbs, tinctures and essential oils. It is known that in ancient Greece of woman rich houses added to the bath rose oil to their skin was smooth and velvety. And Cleopatra took such a bath every day.

The use of essential oils

Modern cosmetology in studies confirmed the faithful folk recipes. Because essential oils have anti-inflammatory effects, strengthen the immune system, tone, rejuvenate and cleanse the skin, helps in the fight against excess weight and cellulite. These substances have on the human body different effects. Therefore, you should select the oil that is best to cope with a certain problem.

How to take a bath with essential oils

To get the greatest benefit from taking a bath with essential oils, it is necessary to know how to apply them correctly.

Do not use too much of the essential oil of aromatic bath. Overdose can lead to skin irritation or headaches. In the large bath is enough 3-4 drops of oil.

It makes no sense to add oil to the bath, because they do not dissolve in water. This bath can even be harmful. Pre-need to add oil to any base and mix thoroughly. As a basis we can take the milk, one cup is enough. Also suitable fine honey, cream, yogurt and sour cream, they should be no more than 3 tablespoons. A volatile oil may be dissolved in the base oil, such as almond. Then the basics you need to take about 10-15 ml. Sometimes, essential oil diluted in sea salt. The efficiency of such baths would be higher, since the salt itself is useful. To do this, take about 4 tablespoons of salt, put in a linen bag (can be wrapped in a cheesecloth) and added to the essential oil. Bag needs a little shake and then lowered into the water.

It is important to observe the procedure and this water temperature. Do not use too much hot water, its temperature should not exceed 38 ° C. Otherwise, the body will increase sweating process that actively interfere with useful substances penetrate into the pores of the body. A good way to check is not too hot water - look in the mirror. If it is misted, then it is diluted with cold water bath.

During the procedure, you should not use other cosmetics - gels, shampoos, soaps, etc. Substances in the composition of these products results lower procedures.

It is important to pre-plan bath. You can not eat close later than 1,5-2 hours before the procedure. The procedure should last no less than 10 and not more than 20 minutes. For longer bathing reverse effect can be achieved. Take baths should be regularly, but not every day. It is best to take a break in 1-2 dnya.Posle procedure is not necessary to wipe dry. After the bath oil still some time to be absorbed into the skin. It is best to wait until the body dries itself or immediately after a bath robe to wear warm. Also, do not after such a procedure to develop active. It is important to give the body to relax. To do this, you can lie down, drink herbal tea, or read a favorite book.

Despite the small dose of essential oil, it has quite a strong therapeutic effect. Therefore, you should be wary of such procedures for people with serious diseases. Such diseases include oncology, angina, epilepsy, diabetes, liver cirrhosis, coronary heart disease, thrombosis, chronic hepatitis, glomerulonephritis, dermatitis, acute inflammation and "weeping" mycoses. Pregnant women should also be careful to use essential oils. This is especially true jasmine, mint, geranium and juniper oils. They have a pretty strong effect on the human body. Not to be mistaken with the choice of oil, you can refer to aromatherapist.

Do not buy synthetic essential oils. They are almost impossible to distinguish from the natural. But oil-in-dark bottle and rather high cost, it is likely to be natural. If the price is about the same, these oils are synthetic nature of the store or pharmacy for all oils.

Recipes baths with essential oils

Baths with essential oils can be used to achieve a cosmetic effect or to calm down. This article lists the most effective prescriptions for different purposes.

When fatigue and irritation to add to the bath 3-4 drops of lavender oil. It helps rejuvenate, relax, improve sleep. Also, when stress and severe stress can use oil of sandalwood, geranium, frankincense and rose. enough to take these oils in an amount of 2-3 drops. If, by contrast, have need to cheer up, it fill the body with energy and strength, here come to the aid of citrus. It is also important not to exceed the dose of 3-4 drops that is enough. Raise the tone will also help oil of rosemary, sage and verbena.

In addition to the emotional stress it is often possible to meet and muscle. This is often with athletes or just people who work hard physically or engaged in the gym. To help your body to relax, to take a bath with a mixture of oil, cinnamon, and lemon balm, ginger and verbena or mint and juniper. Each of the two oils in an amount necessary to take 1-2 drops.

When cold outside, it is very important time to warm up, so as not to get sick. For this is perfect essential oil of thyme, lemon or pine.

When muscle aches and pains in the joints, you can use cedar oil. It helps to relieve the pain.

And if you want a little lift your mood and positive emotions, you can try to add the bath oil of ylang-ylang and sandalwood.

It is known that many essential oils are aphrodisiacs. And that will make a woman more sensual, if not aromatic bath? For this purpose very well suited oil of patchouli, ylang-ylang and neroli. Such bath will not only help to tune in the desired fashion, but also give the skin a pleasant aroma.

Dill Oil. Useful properties and applications of dill oil

Among the green stuff, *dill can be called a leader*, we often add it to salads and hash, sprinkle with him the hot meals and snacks, put in soups and baked goods - nowadays it is present in most recipes. I will not describe dill here: everyone knows about his appearance, smell and taste, but I will tell you about how to get and use the essential oil from this fragrant and useful plant. For a long time, people treated with dill, *kidney disease, stomach and intestines, eye and skin diseases, colds and insomnia*; It has *antiseptic, anti-inflammatory, sedative, diuretic and vasodilator effects, stimulates the production of breast milk in nursing mothers, etc.*

The composition and obtaining of the essential oil from dill.

The dill fruits contain a lot of essential oil, and more often the oil it is produced from them, but it is also present in the green dill too- about 2%. The oil is extracted from the greenery, is characterized by a spicy aroma and softness - it is sometimes used in cosmetics.

The composition of dill oil is unstable and depends on the harvesting time, the conditions of their maturation, and other factors. The dill in the most part consists from terpenes - organic hydrocarbon compounds and their derivatives- carvone - it's present in dill oil in the proportion of 40-50%, and it is that who gives persistent spicy aroma to the dill.

The essential oil is obtained from dill throw steam distillation. Before distillation, the raw material is dried; quality oil should be fluid and easy, completely transparent, colorless or barely with noticeable yellow tint. The aroma of the obtained oil from the fruit, should have the familiar smell of dill: *it is fresh, but warm and sweet, reminiscent of the aroma of cumin* - incidentally, the oil of cumin is combined with dill in mixtures.

The oil from the leaves do smell dill, and is more expensive. When buying oil, you should be sure to learn from what raw material is produced: unscrupulous manufacturers sometimes give out for expensive product oil obtained from a mixture of leaves, fruits and even dill stalks.

Action and uses of dill oil

Dill oil is used in various fields, but about it more often is remembered in connection with food recipes. As a therapeutic agent it was known in ancient times: it was great known to the Egyptians, the Greeks, the Romans and the Jews. We tend to think that the process of distillation was opened by Avicenna in the XI century, but in reality, it appeared much earlier - in ancient Mesopotamia, so that even Roman gladiators, going into the arena, rubbed their bodies with oil from dill, to enhance strength and calm the nerves at the same time. With these goals it is used in modern medicine: it helps to relieve the effects of stress and mental exertion, to gather thoughts and to look at ourselves from another angle. It is interesting that in the Middle Ages, when the Inquisition was raging in Europe, many monks used dill oil to suppress sensuality and subdue the flesh.

The therapeutic effect of the oil depends on what part of the plant it was received from. More expensive oil of dill *improves digestion and appetite, relieves pain and cramps, eliminates fermentation and flatulence, has a diuretic effect, reduces swelling - especially under the eyes, removes toxins, eases infectious and endocrine diseases.* The same oil is prescribed *for bronchial asthma, colds, gout, high blood pressure, disorders of the kidney and heart.*

Dill oil, as does the dill, is the excellent *"assistant"* in nursing mothers - it stimulates the production of milk, but also it is used in the *"irregularities" of the menstrual cycle* - inside and for rubbing. In its composition there are substances that resemble *estrogen* - the female sex hormones, and *increases their production by the body.* Therefore, dill oil is beneficial for *women of any age.*

Rubbing with him is used as *a relaxant and sedative.* With a total body massage oil is rubbed into the following areas: *neck, base of the neck and shoulders, depression on the upper lip, wrists, calves, feet and "solar plexus".*

If twice a week for 10 minutes you will perform a massage of the shoulder girdle with dill oil, you can get *rid of muscle pain and tension; rubbing the calves and the back will help to cope with insomnia.*

Essential dill oil also has *anthelmintic, carminative, laxative, antiseptic, wound healing, antimicrobial action; loosens muscle tension, moisturizes the skin, treats acne rash.*

It is added to *soothing aftershave lotions*, and in dentistry - *a bleaching agent for teeth.* It can be used as *oral freshener*, including all possible mouthwash composition, for purifying the *indoor air*, and *insect repellent.* In the oil burner it is poured 2-3 drops - no more, and for inhalation take 5 drops, and add as much oil chamomile as you can.

Dill oil for weight correction

A great assistant can become essential dill oil, for those *who wish to keep the figure in shape* - it gently but effectively suppresses the *feeling of hunger.* In order to *reduce appetite and speed up the cleansing of the body*, you need to take 6 drops of oil per day by dissolving it in honey: 1 tsp. in the morning, in the 2nd half of the day and at night. Incidentally, the intake is appointed and in other diseases: *oil is not aggressive, so you can even take 3 drops 3 times a day, but no more, and always with honey.*

To correct weight you must do in parallel, aromatic baths and massages. *Bath with essential oils:* dill and cypress oil - 2 drops, rosemary oil - 1 drop, dissolved in an emulsifier (soda, salt, honey), add warm water 36-38 ° C, and take a bath no more than 20 minutes. If desired, you can add a couple of dill oil drops, but not more than 4 in the bath.

Massage with a mixture of oils, which also includes the dill oil, helps to quickly get rid of the *fatty accumulation in problem areas* - the abdomen, thighs, buttocks, etc. In cookery dill oil is used as well as a fresh plant, especially in winter, when there is no green. It is added to any food: soups, salads, meat and fish, to marinades and pastries.

Since dill oil is a natural preservative and spice, it is used in industrial applications: in the alcoholic beverage, food and perfume industry. For example, in the markets can be met, "Dill" soap.

Contraindications for dill oil.

Essential oil of dill is allowed to use to almost everyone, except for pregnant women - in the old days, it is often was used to stimulate the birth; young children under 3 years of age and patients with epilepsy. However, before using it you need to check on individual intolerance, beginning with one drop.

Marigold oil: Properties and applications for hair and face

Marigold oil is considered one of the best base oils used in aromatherapy and other purposes: *for skin, hair, and in the treatment of certain diseases.*

About the medicinal properties of plants - marigold, I need to tell apart, but derived from it oil retains these properties, and the cost of it, compared to other base oils are somewhat higher.

Expensive oil is obtained by the method of maceration - the infusion of dried flowers in warm vegetable oil. This oil is more than a valuable substance, its value is determined by the quantitative content of linoleic acid; the oil have and other fatty acids; carotenoids, triterpenoids - posses *wound-healing, anti-inflammatory, tonic effect,* sterols - *normalize blood cholesterol levels*; phenolic acids - *have a stimulating effect*; bitter sesquiterpene lactones - the substances characterized by high biological activity.

This oil is obtained by another method using carbon dioxide. This method is fairly new, and it provides high-quality oil, with virtually no impurities.

Calendula oil is obtained in liquid form; the color is green when it is poured into a glass bottle, but in blends it gives a greenish-yellow color and eventually becomes almost orange.

Application of calendula oil

Calendula oil is used widely in cosmetics and medicine, externally and even inside; it can also be used in cooking, adding to some dishes.

On the skin, this oil acts like *moisture*, and this becomes noticeable after a couple of minutes after application: try to apply a little oil on the rough skin of hands, and it will become soft, and the cracks will tight. This particular oil protects the hand if you often *work with chemicals or in cold*. Cracks in the heels, it also heals. Because of its quality, calendula oil is used in many skin diseases and problems: *eczema, ulcers, bruise.*

The skin absorption of oil is good, but a little greasy still remains - *you can remove excess fat with a soft cloth.*

At its regular use, *disappears capillary mesh on the skin and face, including - a problem called rosacea.*

For women, this oil helps to solve many problems: it acts as an anti-depressant, resulting in a rate of hormones and normalizes menstrual irregularities. Calendula oil can also be used during pregnancy, as a cosmetic, as well as to lubricate the nipples during breastfeeding.

Calendula oil for the face

The soothing properties of the oil make it the best way to care for *sensitive skin* that often becomes inflamed; in winter, it is administered in a variety of protective composition for facial skin care. Most often, it is added to the finished cream, or used as a mixture with almond oil. In the winter and in the summer Calendula oil helps to *protect the skin*, in winter, it protects us from frostbite, and in summer - from sunburn and insect bites.

- When on the dry and sensitive skin the body oil is applied immediately after a bath or shower - *it is rubbed into the wet skin throw massage movements.*

- You can also take a bath with this oil: in honey, sea salt or soda, dissolve 1 tablespoon of oil and add it to the bath with a water temperature no higher than 38 ° C, and take the bath about 20 minutes. Calendula oils are often used for oily skin, and oil - is no exception. For oily and problematic skin prone to acne and pimples, with him every day doing compresses, or just wipe with it the face.
- In acne do the following mask: Calendula oil (1 tablespoon) mixed with grape seed oil (St. John's wort) (1 tsp) ,chopped pulp from fresh cherries, and aloe juice (2 tablespoons). The mixture is applied to cleansed face for 25 minutes.

When preparing the mixtures of essential oils is recommended to take not pure oil, but mix it with almond or other base oil, and then add essential oil. It is best combined with other essential oils like *chamomile, cypress and lemon.*

Calendula oil for hair

In hair care, calendula oil is also used: In most *irritated scalp, poor hair growth and dandruff.* Due to the fact that the oil is expensive, many are trying to prepare it at home.

- Make it really is possible: it is necessary to put the dried calendula flowers in a glass jar and pour them in any (preferably olive) oil - it have to be covered completely. The jar is kept in a dark place for 2 weeks, shaking it vigorously every 2 days. The oil is then filtered and is used in masks for hair and scalp, and make with him a body massage.
- When the skin is irritated before washing do such a mask: 3 tsp. of Calendula oil is mixed with 1 tsp. jojoba oil, and add the essential oils of rosemary, sage and tea tree - 5 drops. The mixture is rubbed into the scalp, holding a half-hour or an hour, and rinsed with shampoo on hair type. Dry dandruff disappears, and the itching stops.
- For care for the scalp, giving shine to hair and reduce the number of split ends is used cooked oil-based home calendula cream: 6 tablespoons of oil are mixed with other oils: almond and cocoa - 2 tablespoons, shea butter - 3 tablespoons, and put the mix in a glass container in a water bath. Kept in this state for 20 minutes, then pour into a clean and dry glass jar. Store the finished cream in the fridge. The cream is applied not only to the scalp, but also on the entire length of the hair; wash your hair then.
- Besides listed properties, calendula oil also has antibacterial and disinfectant action, and therefore is used for cuts, wounds, burns, frostbite, as well as inside, in certain diseases, as an aid. It can be taken 2 times a day for 1 tablespoon half an hour before a meal - it is not toxic and does not cause poisoning.

For example, it is assigned to the treatment *of liver and biliary tract diseases, gastritis, gastric ulcer and duodenal ulcer, colitis and enterocolitis; as a sedative* - this oil is especially *helpful in climax.*

Buying calendula oil, you have to be careful. The natural oil called Calendula, this is Latin name of the plant. Unless it is written in another language that can be oil for nails, that is a completely different product - oil from African marigold Tagetes. These are different plants, and even the family are different, but they are sometimes confused not only by the sellers but also by the incompetent manufacturers. Sometimes even in one product are two names at once, including their peers, but the plant Tagetes oil is toxic - it contains ketones, and can irritate the skin and mucous membranes. Ketones can also be mutagenic - cause mutations - and carcinogenic action, and therefore, you should learn to distinguish the present calendula oil from non-real one. The method of obtaining the oil from the plant is also important. More expensive than other types is macerate, and it can be used in pure form. The extract obtained via carbon dioxide should be used only in mixtures, and in small concentrations; product obtained using alcohol is much cheaper, but unscrupulous sellers can sell it at the same price to macerate - all you need to know is to avoid becoming a victim of fraud.

Store oil calendula in a dark place in a tightly closed glass vials.

Oils for protection from the sun and tanning (against UV-radiation).UV-protective properties of oils

As a rule, the fair sex is turning to the natural oils in order to obtain quick and even smooth tan. However, we should not forget about the health of the skin. As is known, the solar radiation is divided into three types depending on the wavelength - A, B, and C. A and B rays are directly involved in the tan, but type C rays cause skin damage. They cause cancer and other skin diseases. But the other two types of radiation not only give the skin a beautiful shade, but also heals it, and help deal with a variety of skin disorders, in particular with acne. So all this radiation to not harm the skin, to not sapped and to not old it prematurely, you must use UV-protective agents (from the sun and tanning) - professional or folk. By popular mainly include all kinds of oil - vegetable, basic and essential. Besides protecting the skin from UV rays of type A and B oils help retain moisture in the skin, stimulate the recovery and growth of new cells, nourish the skin and help tan lie more evenly. With these natural remedies, you can not worry about peeling or dry skin. Moreover, the oils penetrate deep into the body and contribute to overall improvement of human health. In India, there are even special oiling procedures to help improve health and restore peace of mind. In addition, the use of oil is very convenient. They can be applied to the skin before swimming, and after exiting the water they remain on the skin. In the market, there are many cosmetic products for specific areas of the body - for the delicate skin of the face, lips, etc. But the oil can be used directly for all.

What oil protect skin from the sun and tanning?

So, what oil is best suited to protect the skin from UV rays? This, above all, is jojoba oil, wheat germ, rosehip, sesame, and cedar. Also good fit calendula oil, avocado, macadamia, argan. For the body, the simplest and most inexpensive option will be already familiar to us the olive oil. This also can be added to ethereal oil to achieve a particular effect. Excellent cope with this task will do walnut oil or St. John's wort. And for the general improvement of the skin, you can use this product, derived from the seeds of wild carrot, green coffee, bergamot, mandarin, and neroli.

How to use the oil to protect from the sun and tanning?

Cooking oils mixture should be done three days before sunbathing. For this purpose, in a 100 ml portion of any of the above natural oils add 30 drops of essential oils. It can be used with one kind of the oil and you could cook the mixture from several suitable oils. For example, you may take 20 drops from essential oil and 10 drops of carrot or bergamot oil. It is important that all the oils must be exclusively natural and of good quality.

The base oil to pour into the bowl of dark glass, then you can add essential oils and cover tightly. During the next three days, the resulting mixture should be stored in a dark place. It must be shaken from time to time. After this time, you need to take a few drops of oil mixture, rub between your palms and rub into the skin. For it is distributed more evenly, the skin can be a little pre-moistened. The resulting amount will be enough for a few times. However, the mixture should be kept no more than 7-10 days.

Also, pay attention to the ingredients of the mixture. For those how are hypersensitive to one of them or by means of pigmentation is better not to use. But in all other cases, it fits perfectly.

Essential oils for tanning.

Essential oils have a very strong influence on the state of the human body because they have an impact on the closest shell biofield - on ester. With fragrances, you can change the mood, get rid of the common cold and even depression. As for the sun, here too, essential oils can help to get a smooth and beautiful skin tone, if applied wisely.

Essential oils can be divided into several types according to the types of effect on sunburn:

-The oils that promote good tan;

-The oils that protect the skin from sunburn;

-Oils that are harmful to the skin during sun exposure;

-Oils used after tanning to improve it or after treatment of burns;

-Oils with no effect on the skin, or neutral.

The last group of essential oils will not be considered, but with the first four groups is very interesting to get to know in order to apply them in everyday life. Especially because the correctly chosen essential oil helps to get smooth and tanned skin tone called bronze. Getting to know the properties of oils will be wiser to start with those that are better not to apply if you are doing sunbathing.

Essential oils that are harmful during tanning.

There are oils with phototoxic properties: they increase the exposure of UV on the skin. As a result of their contact with the skin is reduced cell resistance to the adverse effects of UV rays, and the skin becomes more susceptible to their influence. Therefore, even after a short stay in the strong sunlight, some areas of the skin become inflamed, and can be formed burns. This is due to the fact that under ultraviolet light in the upper skin, tissues produces free radicals which bombard the cells, which is why they die and inflammation occurs. As a result, in the place where the essential oil was applied may appear dark spots, allergic rashes, and inflammation.

To avoid this, before going to the beach you need to carefully read the label on the package of essential oil. And if it says "phototoxicity", or "photosensitive" - it is not suitable for a hike to the beach. It should also be remembered that the essential oils act negatively especially on the exposed skin where they interact directly with ultraviolet rays. After applying phototoxic oils to strong sunlight, the burns can not appear within a day or a few hours - it depends on the interaction of oil with UV power and the degree of sensitivity of the skin. The more sensitive the skin to all kinds of external influences, the more will be this period. Generally, in people with sensitive skin essential oils should be used as gently as possible.

List of phototoxic essential oils is quite long and opened this list the cold-pressed oils that are most exposed to ultraviolet light. In this group, we include: orange oil, bergamot, lemon, thyme, parsley, petit grain, rosemary, angelica, lime, neroli, verbena. If you rubbed your skin with one of this oils and on the skin appeared discomfort and redness, it is necessary to treat the affected areas with a mixture of a dessert spoon of sour cream and 2-3 drops of essential oil of rose. Very well put the compress on the affected skin before bedtime.

Essential oils to get a good tan.

With these oils the procedure is simple: Apply on the skin for a sunbath. However, please know that the essential oil is best used in conjunction with the base oil. It is natural and safe tanning power. For a useful mixture, basic and essential oils are mixed in certain proportions: 100 ml of fatty base oil add 10-15 drops of essential oil or a mixture of bergamot, ylang-ylang, neroli and mandarin. The basis for the tanning of the amplifier is best to take the oil of sesame or avocado.

Essential oils to protect against UV.

The people with sensitive skin often need protection from the sun's rays. It will help the following oils: wheat germ, rosehip, jojoba, avocado, sesame and olive oil.

Oils for skin care after sunbathing.

It often happens that after going to the beach seems to be no burns, but the skin feels somehow uncomfortable. So it should be easy to "calm down." In this case, the aid will come from essential oils of chamomile, rose, cypress, lavender and geranium. Dissolve them better in base oils: apricot pits, almond or jojoba. These funds are not only soothed and soften the skin, but also to consolidate tan.

The use of essential oils for sunburn.

In order to get a nice tan, the skin should be prepared: approximately three days before the hike to the beach, clean the skin from dead cells using a scrub, and at breakfast drink half a glass of carrot juice with cream.

Previous trek to the beach, do not exceed the dosage of oil. It is better to start with the minimum dose, and then the amount of oil can be increased. For a woman's skin needs more concentrated mixture than for men. Light skin is very sensitive to the effects of biologically active substances than dark, so essential oils should be used in the lowest dose and with great caution.

If you use essential oils for tanning constantly - make short breaks. After 2-3 weeks is better to make a week's break. And after the break, the concentration of tanning is better to make more intense, because over time, the skin reaction to the essential oils increases. And again, in the preparation of agents for the skin is better not to mix more than five different types of essential oils.

During pregnancy, the use of essential oils takes place only under the supervision of specialists. With self-application is better to take half the usual dosage. And some oils generally have a contraindication for pregnant women.

Recipes "before and after-sunbath"

To get a good tan:

Mix essential oils: 6 drops of carrot seed and petitgrain and add them to the base oil, which is made up of equal proportions (50 drops) of olive oil, sesame, jojoba and avocado oils. The whole mixture must be vigorously shaken and put on the skin. It can be used for children.

The second recipe: 10 drops of essential oil of ylang-ylang mix with base oils:10 ml of coconut, 5 ml of wheat germ oil and 4 ml of almond. This mixture is used only when the skin tans quickly.

A mixture of oils after sunburn (soothing).

Lavender - 10 drops; Neroli - 10 drops; Blue daisy - 10 drops; Basic jojoba oil - 50 ml.

The second recipe: Lavender - 3 drops; rosemary - 2 drops; sandalwood - 2 drops. As a basis for a soothing mixture is taken 15 ml of any base oil.

The mixture to get rid of wrinkles that appeared after the sunburn.

Essential oil of sweet orange (8 drops) is mixed with carrier oil: hazelnut - 10 ml, almond oil - 4 ml, and wheat germ oil - 2 drops. This mixture is very well applied to the skin in the evening, making it in two stages. The mixture is applied with massaging movements on the limits of the massage lines. There is another good recipe, which can be used from time to time: apply to the skin fresh orange juice for a few minutes, after drying wash away.

Castor oil. Properties and application of castor oil.

Castor oil is derived from castor beans - African plant that botanists refer to the Euphorbiaceae. Grows the shrub or tree, in the north-east of the African continent; can live 10 years and reach a height of 10 meters, but in the northern regions, this plant is not as high - is a shrub, a little more than 2 m, and people often find castor plant an ornamental plant, not having a clue about its benefits and medicinal properties.

Since immemorial times, people know how to get out from the castor plant medicinal oil: the most successful in this were Egyptians - already about 5000 years ago, they used oil, not only in his many religious rituals but also treated diseases with them - they knew about its laxative properties - prepared cosmetics with him. However, it is used as a make-up in their homeland until now: it effectively destroys harmful bacteria, heals small scratches and sores, softens and smoothes the skin. Castor oil is used by local tribes even in cooking: they cook food on it. When heated it collapse toxins and laxative properties are lost; and it has long been used for technical purposes, for processing hides and tanning.

Later Arabs have cultivated varieties of castor beans, in which was a lot of oil; then it became popular in India: they have been treated and prepared with its cosmetics, poured into lamps, etc. Castor spread around the world with explorers and travelers: it came to Europe and America, where natives also learned how to use. Quickly assess the properties of castor oil, the British: they used it not only in cosmetics and perfumes but also as a technical lubricant - it happened just at the time of the Industrial Revolution.

There are two acceptable ways to get oil from it - the seeds of castor beans are used to produce castor oil. Oil of lower quality produced by the method of hot-pressing and more clean and useful is obtained from cold-pressing - just it, is used not only in the manufacture of cosmetics but also in medicine - that is oil that is sold in pharmacies.

Castor oil is composed of fatty acids. Among them, the main one is ricinoleic - about 90% of it. Castor oil also has other fatty acids: oleic and linoleic, and - small quantities - stearic and palmitic.

Properties of castor oil.

Women whose skin is prone to flaking and often weather-beaten may use it, known softening and soothing properties of castor oil, if you have a skin problem or the skin is very dry, this oil can help in most cases. In hair care, castor oil is used more frequently than many other oils, because of its softness; and that it can be used to return the density and luster lashes, today most women know about it.

Since childhood, we know, and that castor oil - colloquially, is actively used in medicine - as a rule, we have heard about the laxative properties of this oil. However, the therapeutic properties are many: it helps to relieve inflammation, softens the skin and mucous membranes, has a restorative effect on the entire body, reduces pain, relieves spasms, etc.

Application of castor oil.

Share details of its application does not work, but at least some health problems can be listed with which it successfully fights.

Castor oil cure skin diseases, wounds, inflammation, bruising, swelling, ulcers, varicose veins, hemorrhoids, eye diseases, gastrointestinal problems; reduces cough; It eliminates constipation, flatulence and stimulates bowel movements; eliminates muscle pain; used in obstetric practice -its help stimulates labor. In pharmacology castor oil is introduced into the composition of the various medications, ointments, and salves - this oil is one of the main components of such a known therapeutic agent, as an ointment Vishnevsky.

Laxative properties of castor oil.

The fact that the castor oil - is the perfect laxative, we know more from the children's books, and it operates as follows. Once in the intestine, it acts on the receptors, increases peristalsis and - after receiving a laxative effect is already apparent after 5-6 hours.

Admission of oil is not very convenient, but before, laxatives were not so much, so it was popular. Adults need to take 15-30 gelatin capsules for half an hour, and children - 10 capsules; it can be taken pure castor oil, 1-2 tablespoons The cause of constipation, oil does not eliminate, so it can not be used for intestinal obstruction.

Treatment with castor oil.

Castor oil treats rectal fissures and hemorrhoids: inserted into the rectum they soaked gauze sponges. For colds and bronchitis oil was also long been used in folk medicine - in combination with turpentine, it is particularly effective.

Gum turpentine produced from turpentine - conifers liquid resin: oil is first heated and then mixed with them in the ratio 2: 1. The mixture is rubbed into the chest and back in the form of heat, massage movements put on warm clothes and lay down under a blanket - of course, it is better to do it at night. If necessary, you can rub again every 3-4 hours - the state will quickly improve. Castor oil is absorbed quickly, and traces on clothes will not appear. When tired and have sore eyes oil can be instilled in them, 1 drop in each eye before going to bed. If you do it during the day, it will temporarily form an oil film.

The use of castor oil for the skin.

At home, in the care of the skin, it is usually mixed 1: 2 or 1: 3 with other natural cosmetic oil base, oil blend is heated in a water bath, and several times a day it is applied to problem areas of the skin.

These oil mixtures can be used to eliminate wrinkles around the eyes: the mixture is gently pierced in the skin at night with fingertips.

You can make it less noticeable the dark spots and freckles, if lubricate them with oil 3-5 times a day, locally. Warts and skin growths can "withdraw" in the same way.

The use of castor oil for hair

Dandruff - it is a problem for many people and for good reason shampoo manufacturers so actively advertise the means to get rid of it. This can be done with the help of castor oil, even if just to rub it into the scalp in front by hook and hold for 25-30 minutes. The scalp hydrated, peeling away, which means "go away" for dandruff.

Castor oil in mixtures.

Take 1 tsp. of castor oil and olive oil, add to it the juice of ½ lemon, and the mixture is applied to the scalp and hair, dandruff amount starts to decrease, and then it will disappear altogether. The hair at the same time become more healthy, shiny and silky.

A very simple recipe: Mix castor oil with calendula tincture, which is in any drugstore. This mixture is also used for half an hour before washing the head - the results are wonderful, if you do it regularly for several months.

If a strong hair loss make a mask with castor oil and alcohol, mixing them in equal parts. The mixture from oil and alcohol is kept on the scalp and hair for at least half an hour and then is washed with shampoo. To stop hair loss, it is necessary to do this procedure for 2 months, 3 times a week.

Contraindications to the use of castor oil (castor) is not so much: hypersensitivity and pregnancy; do not use it and children up to 6 years. Contraindicated its use in case of poisoning with fat-soluble chemicals.

Thyme oil. Treatment and use of essential oil of thyme in cosmetology.

Thyme (thyme) is known for its healing properties since ancient times - about it wrote Dioscorides and Hippocrates, and the inhabitants of the Mediterranean has long been treated with them - this region is considered to be his birthplace. Today, thyme growing in Spain, Central Europe, Russia, Israel, China, Turkey, USA, North Africa; in its nature, there are about 300 species, but thyme - Thymus vulgaris, in aromatherapy is used more often than others. Plant name was translated from the Greek language in different ways: some believe that it comes from the word "thymos" - "fragrance" or "spirit", but in the Greek there is the word "incense" - but essentially it does not change it valour - the scent of thyme is strong, spicy and warm, thanks to thymol and carvacrol - volatile substances from phenolic groups. Monoterpene phenol-thymol is used in the chemical industry, in medicine as an antiseptic, anesthetic and a sedative; in pharmacology - as a preservative; and even in beekeeping - treat diseases of bees. Carvacrol - phenolic monoterpenoid with a pleasant taste and smell, is often used as an antibacterial agent.

These two elements make up the bulk of the essential oil of thyme - about 60%; as it consists of terpene alcohols and monoterpenes, isomeric hydrocarbon terpinene, organic pigments, gum, minerals, bitter tannins, natural ursolic acid, which has expressed a number of medicinal properties; monounsaturated oleic acid, etc.

The composition of essential oils is complicated, and without any special knowledge it is impossible to understand, but in the case of thyme oil you should know something. The fact that thyme – as a plant is highly variable in respect of its chemical composition and structure of its essential oil may vary: it depends on the place of growth, the conditions and acquisition time, etc. If different types of essential oils of other plants do not usually have a sharp differences, different types of thyme oil differs much - in composition, properties, color and aroma. In chemistry there are chemotype concept - essential oil composition depending on the type of plant, and the example of thyme chemotypes difference is clearly visible. The composition of the thyme oil, grown in different climatic conditions, will be different - so much, as if it's different plants, while leaves and flowers, and pollen will be exactly the same. Thyme - this plant have a plurality of chemotypes: its oil can be toxic or irritating, or have powerful medicinal properties, and it is very important to know the chemotype, and - at least in general terms - the main components of its essential oils.

Although in the preparation of oil the irritants are removed from it, even one chemotype oil may have different compositions and have different effects. For example, oil with thymol chemotype can be either a strong irritant and antiseptic, if the plants was harvested in fall, or to have more analgesic effect, if the raw material was collected in the early spring.

The essential oil of thyme

The essential oil of thyme has on the human body a lot of different therapeutic action: tonic, antispasmodic, regenerating, anti-rheumatic, expectorant, diuretic, cardiotonic, anthelmintic, hypertensive, carminative, antibacterial, antiseptic, and others.

Thyme oil relieves insomnia and relieves headaches, improves memory and brain function, helps fight with chronic fatigue syndrome, fatigue and depression, increases the tone of the nervous system as a whole; It improves blood circulation in the capillaries, increases the force of heart contractions, increases the pressure; It leads to normal digestion, eliminates flatulence and intestinal cramps, cleans the digestive tract from harmful microorganisms and improves appetite. In gastroenteritis and oral infections are useful antimicrobial properties of thyme oil, it expels parasites and restore damaged liver cells.

In diseases of the throat and respiratory system, this oil is also effective: for pharyngitis, tonsillitis, laryngitis, flu, colds, sinusitis, coughs, bronchitis, tuberculosis. It stimulates the immune system, helps the body to quickly deal with infections - especially effective against recurrent infections is thymol oil chemotype, although it should be used with great caution.

Actively exerts its therapeutic properties in diseases of the genitourinary system: for inflammation of the fallopian tube and cervix (increases uterine tone and regulates emotional background), cystitis, urinary tract infections and even chlamydiosis - one of the most common diseases among sexually transmitted diseases.

Thyme oil relieves pain and swelling after sports injuries, arthritis, rheumatism, gout, neuritis, myositis and other diseases of the locomotor system; it helps those who want to lose weight.

With the success the thyme oil is used in dermatology. In the treatment of fungal infections especially effective is thymol chemotype; It also relieves itching after insect bites, kills parasites - lice, scabies mites, etc. It helps with dermatitis, psoriasis, eczema, heals ulcers, burns, cuts and wounds.

Oil from thyme for Treatment

Recipes with essential oil of thyme are quite a lot, the most important are here.

In bronchitis, laryngotracheitis, pharyngitis, rhinitis in the room where the patient is, put an aroma lamp with a mixture of oils: thyme - 5 drops, eucalyptus - 3 drops, clove - 2 drops - such a mixture cleans the air, kills germs and prevents the spread of infection.

Appetite can also be adjusted with the thyme oil: for increased appetite before a meal make cold inhalation for 3-5 minutes, dropping 1 drop of oil on a cloth or paper; for decreased appetite help aromatic baths (3-5 drops to a full bath) and the oil burner (3-5 drops per 15 sq. m of the area). In helminthiasis, make microclysters with thyme oil. First oil (2-5 drops) is dissolved in an emulsifier (soda or honey - ½ tsp), and then the mixture is dissolved in 200 ml. of pure water and administered into the rectum. The procedure is repeated 2-3 weeks in a row 2 times a week, combining with the usual enema, in which also add thyme oil - on 1 liter of water.

For internal use the thyme essential oil is taken for insomnia, rheumatism, lung disease, spastic cough, hypotension, anemia, fatigue, etc. At first, it is mixed with the base 1:3, then one drop from this mixture is dissolved in a jam or honey and may be added to the fish or meat dish, to the bread crumb and taken 1-3 times per day. You can drink oil mixed with yogurt, tea, juice and even wine, but you can never take thyme oil on an empty stomach.

Another method used in the treatment of throat diseases is: 2-4 drops of oil of thyme instill in the charcoal tablet, and suck it under the tongue - repeat 2-3 times a day. If the inflammation is severe, you can add to the thyme oil, 2 drops of essential oil from savory.

The use of thyme oil in cosmetics.

As cosmetic essential oil, it is used for cellulite, purifies and tones up flabby or oily skin, eliminates acne.

Thyme oil strengthens the hair and improve their growth - it is especially effective for oily hair. It should be 2 times a week rubbed into the scalp a mixture of thyme and base oil (5 drops per 10-15 ml), add it to your balsam-conditioner (3-5 drops), or just drip a few drops on a comb

Thyme oil is not used for sensitive skin, in liver and kidney diseases, epilepsy, cardiac disorders, hypertension and pregnancy. It is contraindicated in children under 6 years old.

Oil of lemon balm. Properties and application of essential oil of lemon balm

Melissa, or lemon mint - is an perennial plant from the family Labiatae. Lemon balm grows in many regions of the world: Asia and America, North Africa, the Mediterranean and the Middle East, many gardeners also learned how to grow lemon balm on their plots. Melissa is considered a good honey plant – it is liked by bees, and it blooms from July to September, and has the smell of fresh lemon.

Properties of lemon balm oil

Medicinal properties of lemon balm are many, and most of all it is known for its ability to positively influence the nervous system and the brain: it has a stimulating and soothing effect, relieves cramps and dizziness, eliminate tinnitus. In addition, it has antispasmodic, analgesic, diaphoretic, a slight laxative, antiviral, bactericidal, choleretic, carminative, expectorant, antipyretic, wound-healing effect; improves the functioning of the stomach and the heart. The people use it many years ago for painful menstruation, anemia, insomnia, neuralgia, asthma, shortness of breath, poor digestion, colds and others.

A bright lemon scent have the essential oil of lemon balm - it is obtained by steam distillation of all its parts, but most of from the fresh leaves, flowers and stems.

Oils obtained from one plant is very small - only 0.01%, and it is very expensive, so it is more common to find in the sale, oil of lemon balm in a mixture with lemon, commonly used in aromatherapy, but about net oil it is said that it "gives birth to dreams."

As all essential oils, oil of lemon balm have rich and complex composition. It comprises a plurality of esters, monoterpenes, terpene aldehydes and other compounds with strong biological activity. For example, geraniol - terpenoid with the smell of roses, and its related monoterpene myrcene, largely determine the pleasant smell of oil, as well as the plant itself.

Application of lemon balm oil.

In medicine, Melissa oil is used since ancient times: it knew about from ancient Greeks and Romans, and is was used to improve memory, visual acuity, to heal cramps, dysentery and in the treatment of inflammatory diseases.

Soothing and antispasmodic properties of the oil allow its use for insomnia - it acts as a slight sedative; in psychotherapeutic practice it is used to relieve the effects of stress and to restore the energy balance of the body.

Cardiologists recommend it for prevention and for the treatment of uncomplicated heart disease, arrhythmia, shortness of breath and attacks of tachycardia; neurologists also apply it in the treatment of diseases of the autonomic nervous system.

If you take the oil of lemon balm inside, the pressure of blood is reduced, normal heart rate and breathing, also. When you have nervous tension and pressure, you can take a warm (36-37 ° C) bath with lemon balm oil - not more than 5-6 drops.

Essential oil of lemon balm normalize digestion - it soothes gastritis and eliminates bloating; inflammatory diseases of the throat, mouth and respiratory tract.

It reduces headache, fever, stimulates the reproductive system.

Oil of lemon balm in dermatology

In dermatology, it treat fungal infections, boils, eczema, shingles, cold sores; It quickly helps with insect bites - relieves itching and redness. Outwardly it is also used for the treatment of bruises, cuts and wounds, rheumatism, migraines, swollen mammary glands and to repel insects.

When herpes blister appear at first it is necessary to apply a drop of lemon balm oil in its pure form or by mixing it with a drop of any base oil - then these blisters usually do not appear. Apply compresses with balm oil for genital herpes; also in this disease it is taken orally - 2-3 times per day, 1 to 4 drops dissolving then in an coffee spoon with honey and then in a glass of warm water.

Other indications for the reception of oil from lemon balm inside: anemia, painful menstrual periods, depression, memory impairment, pregnancy toxicosis, spasms in asthma, tinnitus, dizziness, fainting, epilepsy, convulsions, insomnia, increased nervous irritability, neuralgia, etc.

You can also take the oil of lemon balm with jam and even mayonnaise and other sauces (5-7 drops per 50 grams), add it to the meat, fish and vegetable dishes.

Essential oil of lemon balm in cosmetology

In cosmetology essential Melissa oil can be used for different purposes, but more often it is used for lip care, oily skin and greasy hair.

Oil of lemon balm for lips

Wound healing properties of lemon balm oil improve the condition of the lips, remove crusts and cracks; in winter it is necessary to add oil to your cream or lip balm - this will protect them from frost and wind. If the lips have lost their brightness and freshness, and have pale red border, it is necessary to put them on a daily basis of any mixture from the base oil (10 ml) and lemon balm essential oil (5 drops).

Oil of lemon balm for the skin

In addition to oily skin, lemon balm oil is excellent for skin aging and sagging, as the balm contains many biologically active substances, causes the skin to tighten and smooth wrinkles. Dry skin also becomes much better after applying balm oil: it moisturizes and nourishes it with oxygen, and removes irritation and flaking. In oily and porous skin well help steam bath. For example, 1 drop of bergamot oil, lemon balm-1 drop, grapefruit-2 drops to 1 liter of water; or - oil of lemon balm, kayaputa, juniper, lemon, marjoram - 1 drop of everything.

Oil of lemon balm enriched cosmetic - 5-8 drops per 15 ml; use a mixture of oil: 10 ml of base oil, 1-3 drops of essential oils - such as lemon balm- 1 drop, 2 drop of grapefruit, 3 drops bergamot - this mixture is suitable for oily skin.

Effective mask for oily skin with enlarged pores: mix in equal parts- wheat germ oil, grape seed oil, cosmetic clay and spirulina powder, to 5 ml of this mixture add 3 drops of lemon balm oil and apply on the face, trying to impose on the areas with enlarged pores in thicker layer. Hold for 5 minutes and wash off with water at room temperature.

Cosmetic ice with lemon balm oil tones and revitalizes the skin of any type. It is necessary to mix 2 drops of oil with cosmetic cream or honey, then dissolve in a glass of water, pour into molds and freeze. Use in morning and evening, wipe the face, neck and décolleté.

Oil of lemon balm for hair

In greasy hair and dandruff, to your shampoo add a few drops of lemon balm oil. If you wash your hair with such a composition for 1.5 months, the hair will become healthy and strong.

With oil of lemon balm you can make a mask for oily hair and scalp massage: it will reduce the activity of the sebaceous glands and the hair will no longer stick together. The result can be obtained more quickly if the oil is mixed with essential oils of lemon balm, fir, cedar, lavender, sage, thyme, lemon, etc., as base oil is good to use burdock.

The good masks are derived from balsam for oily hair: added thereto 5-7 ml of macadamia oil, and 5-7 drops of lemon balm oil, mixed with cosmetic clay and everything is thoroughly mixed and applied on hair partings on the scalp. Cover head with foil and heat with a thick towel, hold for 10-15 minutes and wash off with warm water.

For oily hair, you can add 8-10 drops of lemon balm oil in your hair conditioner.

Baths with lemon balm oil

Body Spa is not only improve the skin condition, but also to relieve the general tension. In warm (37-38 ° C) water bath is added oil of lemon balm (5 drops), dissolving it in the sea salt, cream or honey. The bath can be taken no more than 20 minutes and wipe dry with a towel. For sensitive skin are enough 3-4 drops of oil, otherwise you can get severe burns.

In weary skin in a bath is added melissa and neroli oil - 2 drops of each, and oil from rosewood - 3 drops.

Do not apply oil if you are hypersensitive, during pregnancy. You can not use it continuously for more than 2 weeks. Not recommended for people whose work is connected with the use of voice (singers, speakers, etc..), as it may cause a sore throat. In excess doses, the oil can cause lethargy and drowsiness.

Cocoa butter: composition and properties of the treatment.

Your favorite product – is chocolate, as we know it is prepared from cocoa beans and is considered to be the most delicious sweet - one that "melts in your mouth, not in your hand." In this product should be a lot of natural cocoa butter - according to the rules, it should be dipped in chocolate, but the producers, seeking to save mnoney, add cheaper vegetable oils: coconut, palm and others.

Cacao oil

Cocoa oil have not only excellent taste: it is very nutritious, useful and healing - it has long been used not only in cooking and cosmetics, but also treat many diseases, using it as an outward and inward.

Cosmetologists are very fond of this oil, and it is said that the more efficient can only be called shea oil, that since ancient times helps women to prolong youth and maintain beauty.

Cocoa beans, people used to call the seeds of the tree of chocolate, although it is not quite right - but the name somehow stuck. First, the seeds should undergo fermentation process - the so-called soaking in special tanks, after which the pulp is easily separated from the shells. The fermented seeds are dried and roasted - shell becomes brittle and is removed, and the seeds are ground and extracted from them, oil - by hot pressing. The oil is immediately filtered, and then poured into molds, and then it freezes: it becomes quite hard substance of light yellow color with pleasant delicate scent of chocolate. At room temperature (at least at 18 ° C) cocoa butter is always hard, but it melts quickly and easily - it is necessary to heat it up to 30-40 ° C, to store it, and then use in cosmetic and medicinal purposes is very conveniently.

The composition of cocoa butter

In general terms the composition of cocoa butter is short - it consists of a triglyceride - glycerine and fatty acid-esters: oleic, stearic, palmitic, linoleic, etc. The cocoa oil contain also many of the amino acids, so it is chemically stable and did not oxidize - if it is a part of cosmetics, its shelf life increases.

The properties of the cocoa butter

Thanks to these fatty acids, cocoa butter has a pronounced skin regenerating effect, and is suitable for all types of skin - even children's skin gives no allergic reactions, and beautifully softens and protects. It smoothes and heals defects - traces of burns, scars and roughness, eliminates stretch marks and dark spots. It helps in the treatment of dermatitis, eczema and other skin problems.

The rich mineral composition - calcium, iron, magnesium, chromium, iodine, etc., allows to use the cocoa butter as a therapeutic and preventive agent for many diseases - for example, it strengthens the walls of blood vessels, prevents the development of atherosclerosis, varicose veins, etc. If you use it regularly, can improve cerebral blood flow, significantly reduce the risk of heart attack, allergies, stomach ulcers and even cancer.

Research conducted by the Latin American scientists have shown that cocoa butter reduces the risk of cancer by 15 times - for this it is necessary to regularly use for 5-10 years.

British scientists have also shown that this oil is more effective for the treatment of cough than many medicines: it has a natural theobromine, so it works gently, but quickly, and does not cause side effects as synthetic drugs.

Cocoa butter treatment

Preparing popular cough medicine with just 1-½ tsp. of cocoa butter added to the beaker of hot milk, stir and drink - so doing 3-4 times a day and soon cough retreats. This tool not only helps with bronchitis and acute respiratory viral infections, pneumonia, asthma. Bronchitis, except ingestion, should be treat with a cocoa butter massage for chest - it speeds up the healing process.

During epidemics of influenza and other acute respiratory viral infections, nasal mucosa should be lubricated with oil of cocoa: it will soften and protect it, creating a barrier to viruses - because all infections are transmitted by airborne droplets.

In tuberculosis, pneumonia and tonsillitis take a mixture of cocoa butter (10 parts) with propolis (1 part). Melt butter in a water bath by adding crushed propolis, and stirring constantly; then remove and continue to stir until the mixture has cooled. Take 3 times a day, ½ tbsp.. one hour before meals.

In atherosclerosis cocoa butter is taken before breakfast and dinner, 15 minutes before meals, ½ tsp.. It cleanse the body from "bad" cholesterol, preventing it deposited on vessel walls.

As a cholagogue, cocoa butter is used for cholecystitis, drink in the morning 1 tablespoon on an empty stomach, melt in a water bath, then put a heating pad under the right side and then lay down in bed for 1.5-2 hours. It is enough to do it at least once a week - in the output when it is not necessary to go to work.

Cocoa butter (1 teaspoon) in combination with the sea-buckthorn (10 drops) for cervical erosion: with this mixture impregnate a swab and injected deep into the vagina at night - the procedure is repeated daily for 2-3 weeks.

Cocoa butter in the home cosmetics

Home Cosmetics, safe and effective, with cocoa butter can be cooked a lot - like masks, ointments, creams, balms; you can simply add it to your cream for face, body and hair.

For all skin types, except oily and problematic, suitable scrub with cocoa butter. Solid oil (2 tablespoons), put in a small container in a water bath, melt and add honey (1 tablespoon), stir, remove, and immediately add oatmeal and raw ground nuts (1 tsp.). You can take the walnuts, almonds, hazelnuts, cashews, etc. Everything is again stirred and allowed to cool, then applied a bit of the mixture on a wet face and gently massage in a circular motion for 2-3 minutes. It is possible to roll small balls of the mixture and use them a few times - they are easy to melt in your hands and apply to the skin. If you have dry and flaky skin, facial scrub is particularly helpful - it makes it smooth and soft.

Withering skin is animated with cocoa butter, grape seed and aloe mask. In one tablespoon of grape oil add one tsp. of melted cocoa butter, mix, add 1 tablespoon of chopped pulp of aloe, mix again, and in the heat form put on the face. Hold for 15-20 minutes and wash off with warm, then cool water. The mask has moisturizing, vitaminizing, slight astringent and rejuvenating effect.

For daily care for oily skin, you can prepare homemade cream with cocoa butter (2 tablespoon) canola or almond oil (90 ml), lavender essential oil (3 drops), and basil or rosemary tea (4 tablespoon). The ingredients are thoroughly blended and mixture is keep in a glass jar and store in the refrigerator.

Like above prepared and stored cream for sensitive skin: cocoa butter (2 tablespoons), sunflower oil (90 ml), sandalwood essential oil (5-6 drops), infusion of tea rose (4 tablespoons).

Hair also "like" mixture from cocoa butter: it moisturizes and strengthens them, return them to shine and prevents hair loss.

Firming mask with cocoa butter (2-3 tablespoons) and rosemary broth - it should be done 10-12 times, 2 times a week. Melted butter is mixed with warm broth, rub mixture into the hair roots and distribute throughout their length, cover with foil and keep the head for 2-3 hours. Wash your hair with your shampoo. That hair stopped falling out, it is necessary 2-3 times a week to make a mask with cocoa butter, and burdock (1 tablespoon), raw egg yolk and yogurt (1 tablespoon). To the heated cocoa butter are added burdock, then the egg yolk and yogurt, mixed thoroughly and the mixture is applied to the hair roots and scalp. Cover head with foil and a thick towel, hold 1.5-2 hours and wash your hair with shampoo. Total need to do 12-16 procedures.

Cocoa butter is ideal for protecting the skin from frost and wind - in winter it is applied to the face before going out; from heat and UV rays, it also protects before you go sunbathing, apply oil all over the body and the skin does not dry up.

Great care for eyelids and lips - it may be applied in pure form or blended with other oils - for example, sesame or almond.

Eyelashes and eyebrows with it regular use are also strengthened: become smooth, healthy and thick.

Contraindications to the use of cocoa butter are not enough: outwardly and inwardly - idiosyncrasy; Only inside - increased nervous irritability and insomnia, but it can be used in the daytime.

Celandine oil: composition, useful properties. The use and treatment of essential oil of celandine.

Celandine as a remedy in folk medicine is used for a long time, we all know about its medicinal properties in the treatment of various skin diseases. Even its name speaks for itself: "celandine" means "clean body" or "clean skin". By this seemingly nondescript plant, our ancestors have always been treated with great respect, because it gets rid of many ailments, in children and adults. Useful properties have not only the plant itself, but also its oil.

Celandine oil has a purifying effect on the skin, relieving people from various skin diseases. Often it is used in pimples, irritation, acne, etc. One advantage of this oil - is the possibility of its application in the treatment of infants. As is known, toddlers often suffer from skin irritations. Here celandine oil comes in, gently and painlessly soothing the skin and removing redness. Simply rub the problem areas of the skin and after a while the irritation will disappear.

The composition of the oil of celandine

In celandine oil composition are many useful substances, healing, namely: alkaloydy, carotene, vitamin C, saponins, flavonoids, bitter, organic acids (malic, citric, and succinic acid) and a resinous material.

Among the alkaloids contain also: chelidonine and sanguinarine. Chelidonine has properties similar to morphine, with a very strong local anesthetic effects. It promotes inhibition of the nervous system and reduce the sensitivity of the body. Sanguinarine has the same property, but in addition it also affects the digestive system, stimulating bowel activity and salivation. Also, this substance has analgesic property.

Useful properties of celandine

Celandine oil is capable of exerting anti-bacterial, anti-inflammatory, analgesic, wound healing and anti-allergic effect. Doctors often recommend the use of this agent for the treatment of various skin diseases. For example, it can be used to get rid of psoriatic plaques, corns, skin tuberculosis, etc. Of course, it has a beneficial effect on the skin and under such common diseases as acne vulgaris, furunculosis, microbial eczema, seborrhea, etc.

An interesting fact is that celandine oil acts even in an environment that has had time to develop resistance to antibiotics. *Sometimes folk remedy becomes more effective therapeutic drug.*

In diseases accompanied by pruritus, also come to the aid the oil of celandine. It effectively soothes the skin, removing the itching. It also helps with polyps and papillomatosis. Also, celandine oil can be used as an antifungal and antiviral agent. Therefore, it can also be used as a cure for herpes, warts, and even stripping. Thanks to the antibacterial properties of this tool is sometimes used in dentistry and in the treatment of periodontal disease.

The use of celandine oil

Celandine Oil can be purchased at the pharmacy. However, it is possible to cook it independently. To do this, you must first collect the raw materials. To prepare the oils typically use only the upper part of the plant, roots are not needed. Collect the celandine grass need during the flowering period, when the bushes are covered with small yellow flowers. It is best to go on the search for raw materials in May or June. To confuse celandine with other plants is difficult. If you cut it, the yellow liquid will appear on the stem. If you apply it on the skin, then over time it darkens and becomes brown. Celandine grows everywhere - in parks, gardens, in the woods. Villagers usually do not have to look for him. This plant is like a weed surrounding fences, front gardens and kitchen gardens. It is also important to collect celandine in dry weather, and the need to choose plants that are in the shade. Then the raw material would have the most powerful healing properties. Traditional medicine also says that the most useful raw materials from celandine is obtained by collecting it at the growing moon. Cut plants, departing from the soil about 10 cm. This is best to do with gloves, it is important to ensure that the plant juice did not get into eyes. *You must remember that its juice in its pure form has toxic properties.*

After collecting, the plants can be cut into several pieces and spread out to dry. The place for this procedure should be dry, well-ventilated and non-solar. For celandine not accidentally began to rot, it can be from time to time shift or flip. When raw materials become completely dry, you can fold it into a linen bag and use as needed, because from dried celandine can be done not only oil, but also tinctures, decoctions. During the drying and storage, we need to make sure that children are not tried to eat celandine. *This is very dangerous for their health.*

To prepare the oil, dried celandine grass should be put in a glass bowl and pour the oil on top. You can also use normal sunflower oil, but it is best suitable apricot, almond and peach oil. In the case of sunflower oil it is best to preheat it on water bath for 1-2 hours. And, of course, use of refined oil is not necessary. Oil is necessary to fill so that the above raw material must form a layer of a few centimeters of oil. The resulting mixture should be put in a dark, warm place for 1 hour. After that, the dishes can be rearranged in a cool place and leave it for a week. From time to time it is necessary to shake the contents of the dishes. And at the end of the period it should drain and add to the resulting oil, the same amount of ordinary pure oil. Healing celandine oil is ready for use. Keep it in a glass container, preferably in a dark place. The resulting celandine oil is often used in cosmetics. It is particularly effective against acne. However, we must bear in mind that temporary rash can become greater when you use it. But soon they will disappear completely.

For different purposes celandine oil is used in different ways. To remove the wart or callus is necessary to put a little oil on the affected skin several times a day. The treatment period may be different, it is possible to stop at the desired result. In acne or irritation, oil is applied on problem areas for 10-15 minutes and then gently is removed.

Celandine oil has almost no contraindications. It can even be used for treating young children. However, preliminary make sure that you have tolerance to celandine oil. It is also worth considering that the safety of celandine oil does not extend to the plant itself. Celandine juice has quite a sharp effect on the skin, can cause a burn.

Essential oil from Frankincense: application, useful properties and composition.

Essential oils are gaining increasing popularity. We are willing to use them in cosmetics, aromatherapy and treatment of various diseases. It's all in a unique composition of essential oils, thanks to which they have different medicinal properties. Such therapeutic agents include essential oil from incense (frankincense).

Frankincense - a small tree that grows primarily in North Africa and some other countries of the Arab world, and collect it as follows: first, on the bark of a tree make an incision from which the gradually is released liquid resin. Over time, it hardens and becomes a viscous material having amber or orange-brown. And itself oil is obtained by steam distillation. Our ancestors did not make incisions in the bark, they collected liquid remedy that stands out naturally. But over time, the essential oil of incense became so popular that it was necessary to extract the resin on an industrial scale.

Frankincense oil - a pale yellow liquid, sometimes has a greenish tint. Its flavor is a reminiscent of camphor, very warm and sweet.

Frankincense resin is used from antiquity. In India, China and other countries, it was used as incense, and Christians used it, too. The ancients believed that incense is able to drive out evil spirits. In fact, recent studies show that incense aroma helps calm the nervous system, entering into a state of prayer or meditation. In ancient times incense resin was not only used for rituals and ceremonies, but also in the manufacture of cosmetics. Also, it can help treat some diseases and was used in embalming.

The composition of essential oils of frankincense

The composition of Frankincense oil includes a wide variety of materials, thanks to which it has unique healing properties and unique aroma. Among them - the alpha-pinene, beta-pinene, verbenone, alpha pinokarveol, limonene, sabine, myrcene, beta-elements, the alpha and beta celine intsesola, cadinene, cymene, triene alcohol.

The beneficial properties of essential oils of frankincense

One of the important properties of frankincense oil - wound healing, it can be used for various wounds, cuts, etc. It also greatly helps with inflammation of the respiratory system, soothes the mucous membrane, can relieve asthma, cough, runny nose, and shortness of breath. The use of frankincense oil is to optimize the work of the respiratory system, saturate the tissues with oxygen. In general, the essential oil of frankincense promotes regeneration and tissue repair.

Frankincense oil helps to normalize the work of endocrine glands, thereby setting up the whole body. He also has a beneficial effect on the digestive system by adjusting the activity of the stomach and intestines. Particularly fond of frankincense oil for women. After all, it greatly helps to reduce isolation during menstruation, it helps to stop uterine bleeding. It may be used it in the period of pregnancy and childbirth. After all, it is perfectly soothes and helps get rid of depression.

Frankincense oil is used not only for internal use, but also externally. It has a rejuvenating effect on the skin, smoothing wrinkles and tightening the skin. Also, it perfectly removes various inflammations, soothes the skin, makes the complexion smoother and clear pores. It is to known that people who use this oil from a young age, facing with the problem of aging is significantly later than others. Also it is used in dry brittle hair and nails. It helps to restore their natural beauty and health.

Use of frankincense fragrance

It contributes to the pacification, get rid of stress and insomnia, it helps overcome the effects of burnout. In the eastern medicine it is believed that incense aroma helps to restore and strengthen the protection of human energy, and controls the flow of thoughts and align your breath. It promotes peace and enlightenment, perfect for meditation. Also, it is an aphrodisiac, enhances the sensuality in the relationship of men and women, increases libido.

The use of essential oil of frankincense

In folk medicine, frankincense oil is often used for the treatment of respiratory organs. It has established itself as an excellent remedy for asthma. Also, it is quite effective for inflammation of the bronchi, lungs and nasopharynx. Frankincense essential oil is used as a soothing cough, expectorant, cleansing and oxygenates means.

Also it is used for getting rid of seizures, as it promotes circulation. Apply oil from incense in diseases of the bladder, so it great fights inflammation. It is known that it is effective for headaches and dizziness.

Use essential oils from incense for the regulation of the lymphatic system. This oil helps to reduce inflammation and removal of lymph nodes, provides normal lymphatic drainage, removing the body from the stagnant lymph. Often it is used to facilitate the flow of menstruation in women, frankincense oil helps reduce the amount of emissions and helps to get rid of the pain. More years ago healers used it to improve the digestive organs, rheumatic pain, infections of the genitourinary system, skin, colds, and even sexually transmitted diseases. Recipes that they use came up to our days. In virtue of it antiseptic action, incense oil it is used in the manufacture of cosmetics for all skin types. It is often added to creams, masks and serum for problem skin. This oil is used in the treatment of acne to reduce inflammation. Due to the effects of rejuvenating, frankincense oil as it is added to a cream and a mask for aging skin. It also has a bleaching property. Use of a small incense oil helps to remove wrinkles and even small scars, make the skin more elastic. With spot-on it copes with boils, sores, wounds and other skin disorders. It is not necessary to seek funds from the oil of incense, you can enrich your favorite cosmetics for skin and hair care products alone. For this, in 10 ml of base is usually added 5-7 drops of oil.

Indispensable incense oil is in the treatment of dry and brittle hair. You can also add essential oil of frankincense in shampoo, conditioner or mask, and after some time the hair will become silky, shiny and healthy. Also, this tool excels with dandruff, hair loss and stimulate their growth.

The scent of incense is particularly popular with people who practice meditation. However, anyone who wants to relax after a hard day, relieve stress and prepare to sleep, may use this oil. Often it is recommended to use in sexual dysfunction. To use correct frankincense oil, is enough to drip 3-5 drops in aroma lamp and light in it for 5-10 minutes. It can also be used in making a relaxing bath, adding it in water in the same amount.

The essential oil of myrrh. The composition, properties and applications of myrrh oil.

The essential oil of myrrh is obtained from Commifora Abyssinian or myrrh. Therefore, it is called kommiforovym oil. And the plant from which it is prepared the raw material for its production, also called myrrh or Balsam tree. Myrrh trees grow in northeastern Africa, in the Arab East, especially a lot of it in the southern part of the Arabian Peninsula.

The trunks of these trees contains myrrh oleoresins, which has a pale yellow color, and when it is dry becomes more viscous and becomes dark brown. To collect this resin, incisions are made on the bark of trees. When it freezes and becomes a consistency similar to wax, steam distillation is used to obtain essential oil of myrrh. Myrrh resin has a balsamic, bitter and pungent smell, it is also called bitter myrrh.

The composition of the essential oil of myrrh

The composition of essential oil of myrrh includes substances such as linalool, beta-bourbonen, elemen, the alpha-santal, caryophyllene, humulene, cadinene, celine, germakren D, kurtser, elemol and bisabolen. Also, it contains isomers of lindestrena - a substance through which myrrh has a sharp bitter flavor.

The properties of essential oil of myrrh

Essential oil from Myrrh is an liquid oil, which may have a pale-yellow, green-yellow or yellowish-brown color. It has quite a pungent smell, bitter, spicy with camphor and myrrh tone. Oil has antimicrobial, anti-inflammatory, antifungal, wound healing and analgesic effect. The oil has a beneficial effect on the skin, eliminating inflammation. It is also able to strengthen hair. Also it can be used as a diaphoretic, diuretic, expectorant, deodorant, carminative, balsamic, cooling and astringent.

Myrrh oil is an excellent tool in the rehabilitation of patients, can speed recovery after serious diseases and injuries, operations etc. It has a beneficial effect on the immune system, improves circulation, helps with swollen lymph nodes. Also myrrh oil has a beneficial effect on the digestive system: it stimulates the stomach, normalizes the secretion of gastric juice, neutralize bad breath.

The essential oil of myrrh is an aphrodisiac, that is, increases sexual desire in both men and women, making a person more sensual. It is useful especially for women. Myrrh oil can relieve menstrual flow, normalizes the work of the uterus, reduces pain during menstruation.

Useful is and the aroma of myrrh oil. It has a powerful effect on the emotional background of the person. Myrrh oil is able to calm and get rid of depression. This fragrance is designed for state of meditation, it helps to distract from daily problems, to lighten the mood. Also, it helps in fatigue, has an invigorating effect, fills the power.

It has a beneficial effect on human skin. It prevents skin aging, rejuvenating, tightening and reviving the skin, removes wrinkles and even helps dissolve scars and stretch marks. Also oil of myrrh – is a great regenerating agent which promotes the healing of wounds and sores, allergies and neuro-humoral dermatitis.

The use of myrrh oil

Of course, myrrh oil is often used in cosmetics. It is added to a variety of means to care for the face, body and hair. You can also may do with oil of myrrh for cosmetics popular recipes by mixing it with other essential oils and natural products. Use it for skin rejuvenation, get rid of scars, ulcers, stretch marks. It is also used in skin problems, prone to inflammation, rashes and infiltrates. With regular use of it, skin becomes matte and velvety, improves its color. Also, it helps with hair loss. The essential oil of myrrh activates the hair follicle, thereby strengthening the hair, making them thicker and healthier.

To enrich the cream, shampoo, tonic or other cosmetics, is enough to add in 10 ml of base about 7 drops of myrrh oil. Also you can make compresses with this oil. How to do this, in 1 cup of warm water dissolve 5-7 drops of myrrh oil. For application, 5 myrrh oil droplets are mixed with 3 drops of orange oil and added to 10 ml of base oil (olive oil, linseed oil, jojoba oil, grape seed oil). With this substance you may do massage. For this purpose, in 10 ml of base oil add 5-7 drops of myrrh oil. In order to make cosmetic and bath with oil of myrrh do this: 5-7 oil drops are mixed with 50 ml of milk, honey solution, serum, moth marine and add to water.

In aromatherapy essential oil of myrrh is used for insomnia, nervous exhaustion, depression, lowering the tone of the nervous system to recover after a heavy stress - physical or mental. In the aroma lamp is enough to add 5-7 drops of myrrh oil.

Also with oil of myrrh make inhalation for treatment of infections of the upper respiratory tract and throat. Especially when you cough or suffer from runny nose, sore throat, bronchitis, catarrh, sore throat, loss of voice, hoarseness, and sinusitis.

Use it, and in diseases of the mouth. Myrrh oil is effective in bleeding gums, inflammation, stomatitis, gingivitis, periodontitis and ulcers. Also, medicine oil of myrrh is used to treat digestive system. Thus, according to research, helps to get rid of diseases such as flatulence, diarrhea, dyspepsia. Oil of myrrh also helps in hemorrhoids.

Myrrh oil can be used in women's diseases associated with gynecology and urology. It works particularly effectively in menstruation pain.

In addition to medical and cosmetic use of the essential oil of myrrh, it is also used in industry. It is a component of some pharmaceutical drugs, food, alcohol, cosmetics and perfume products.

It has virtually no contraindications. With care it is necessary to treat pregnant women, and people with individual intolerance to any substance included in its composition.

Thistle oil. Application properties and contraindications for thistle oil.

Thistle has long been widely used in the pharmaceutical and medicine, and it is considered a strong drug. It may also be called an effective tool that is used to prevent many diseases. Thanks to its numerous beneficial properties, it is very widely used in folk medicine. From a medical point of view, the most valuable is the thistle oil, it can be used both internally and externally. The oil is cold pressed from the seeds of milk thistle. Externally, it is an oily liquid, which has a yellowish-green color and pleasant specific smell and taste.

The use of thistle oil

It should be noted that the healing properties of milk thistle in people were known from antiquity. The first mention of it can be found in the writings of the ancient physicians. Now the use of this plant is allowed by official medicine in many countries.

Thistle oil is indicated in people recovering from liver disease, as well as those who oppose alcohol or drugs. This oil is recommended after a course of chemotherapy or radiotherapy.

Thistle oil is able to eliminate the side effects of medication, which adversely affect the liver. This oil is very helpful in diseases of the intestine, liver and stomach. *Indications for the use of this oil are:* cirrhosis and fatty liver, hepatitis, acute and chronic gastritis, gastric and duodenal ulcers, biliary dyskinesia. Thistle oil is also indicated in periodontitis and stomatitis.

Thistle oil is widely used by dermatologists. It is useful for many types of dermatitis, allergic skin diseases, hair loss, psoriasis, burns, skin, diaper rash, vitiligo, acne vulgaris, lichen planus, and others.

Thistle oil is used in case of problems with the cardiovascular system, diseases of the ear, nose and throat; as well as in women's diseases.

Contraindications for thistle oil

Importantly, the use of milk thistle oil has no contraindications, it is absolutely harmless. However, in case of serious illness, it is better to discuss the use and dosage of milk thistle oil with your doctor.

Thistle oil properties

The main active ingredient of this plant is silymarin. In the thistle oil, there are 12 kinds of silymarin. These substances help to strengthen cell membranes, especially in the liver cells. As we know, first is the liver, who takes the brunt of the effects of various toxic substances. Therefore, liver health is very important. And silymarin exerts beneficial effects on the human liver, strengthening and regenerating its cells. This oil activates the metabolism, helps burn fat. It has a choleretic effect. Because the development of sufficient bile is simply necessary for the normal digestive process in the body. Therefore, milk thistle has a positive effect on digestion.

Milk thistle oil is rich in liposoluble vitamins A, D, E, F. Vitamin F represents a combination of polyunsaturated fatty acids. Due to their content, this oil has anti-sclerotic effect. These substances are very important for the human cardiovascular system. They reduce the level of harmful cholesterol in the blood by inhibiting its deposition on the walls of blood vessels. Thus, polyunsaturated fatty acids prevent such terrible phenomena such as atherosclerosis, heart attack and stroke. These substances are needed for normal functioning of our brain. Thistle oil has anti-inflammatory, anti-ulcer effect, it is also an effective hepatoprotective. This oil can strengthen the immune system and increase overall resistance to various diseases.

1. Chlorophyll activates the metabolic processes occurring in the cells of the body. This substance is able to exert on the tissue rejuvenating effect. It stimulates the metabolism in the liver and heart muscle, it is necessary to carry out redox reactions in cells.
2. Tocopherols help to protect our body from the effects of the factors that cause the development of cancer. These substances also prevent premature aging and maintain its reproductive function.
3. Carotenoids have antiallergic effects. They are necessary for normal metabolism in the liver and heart muscle. Carotene is necessary for the retina, and as a growth factor.

The thistle oil has a significant amount of vitamins E and A, which are powerful antioxidants. They protect the body from premature aging, as well as the development of malignant processes in it. Vitamin E is necessary for normal functioning of our reproductive system. These vitamins have a positive effect on the condition of our skin and eyes, prevent the development of inflammatory processes. It contains and vitamin

D, which is needed by the body for the full assimilation of phosphorus and calcium. It enhances immunity and normal functioning of the heart, blood vessels and the thyroid gland.

Thistle oil contains large amounts of minerals, such as zinc, selenium, magnesium and manganese. These substances are responsible for the normal synthesis of the hormone insulin by the pancreas. Vitamins B are essential for the full activity of the brain, nervous, cardiovascular, endocrine and muscular systems of the human body.

Thistle oil in cosmetics

Excellent results provides a face and neck massage with oil of milk thistle. This massage is recommended after evening washing and it should be left on all night on face. Conveniently, this oil can be used in any type of facial skin. It nourishes the skin with vitamins, nourishes and moisturizes, promotes skin rejuvenation. The use of this oil makes it possible to improve the protective function of the skin, improve complexion, make the skin more supple and elastic. It accelerates blood circulation in the skin, which smoothes shallow wrinkles on the face. If you lubricate the skin with this oil before going out, it effectively protects it from frostbite, chapping, as well as from the negative effects of sunlight.

You can use milk thistle oil on a daily basis, not only in pure form but also mix it with other oils - olive, almond, etc. It soothes the skin and prevents acne.

The oil prevents the development of varicose veins by strengthening the walls of the subcutaneous capillaries. It also contributes to prevention of cellulite, so it is often used in anti-cellulite massage procedure.

In addition, this type of oil helps to strengthen nails and hair, promotes their growth.

Rosehip oil: structure, properties, application, treatment. Rosehip oil in cosmetology: for the face, décolleté, hair and stretch marks.

Rosehip oil (Oleum Rosae), also known popularly as "sunshine liquid " has a rather complicated production technology. To cook it is used pre-dried seeds of wild rose hips, which are then ground and by hot extraction with organic solvents is obtained the oily liquid.

Rosehip oil: Composition

Rosehip oil has a specific unobtrusive flavor and bitter taste. And depending on the type of plant and the place of it growth, rosehip oil can vary in color from pinkish-golden to bright orange or even brown.

The chemical composition of rosehip oil contained different saturated and unsaturated fatty acids including linoleic, linolenic, oleic, stearic, myristic and palmitic acid. In addition, fatty oil - the main component of the seeds, rich in carotene (vitamin A), tocopherol (vitamin E) and contains a sufficient amount of vitamins C and F. Such trace elements such as copper, molybdenum, strontium and macroelements as iron, calcium, magnesium, manganese, phosphorus, also are part of rosehip oil.

Rosehip oil: Properties, use and treatment

First of all, rosehip oil - is an excellent natural cholagogue. Its useful to use in cholecystitis, hepatitis and other diseases associated with the deterioration of bile secretion process.

Positively, it influences the secretion of gastric juice, and therefore, it is recommended in various forms of gastritis.

It is believed that when it is used regularly, rosehip oil decrease in blood cholesterol levels. This is, firstly, prevention of cardiovascular disease, and secondly, helps in the fight against excess weight. Rosehip oil is also useful for patients suffering from atherosclerosis, as it strengthens the walls of blood vessels and prevents the formation of atherosclerotic plaques, while contributing resorption.

In addition, oil is used as a means of fortifying and multivitamin in infectious diseases, vitamin deficiency, bleeding, burns and frostbite. In the latter two cases, rosehip oil can be used both internally and externally due to its unique ability to accelerate the healing of wounds, thermal burns, and even radiation injuries. The wound healing properties of the oil should also be remembered in cases of stomatitis and gingivitis. It will not only contribute to a more rapid recovery, but also increases the protective properties of the oral mucosa.

Rosehip oil is often recommended as nose drops in rhinitis, pharyngitis and other diseases of the mucous membranes of the nose and throat. In some cases, instead of instillation, in the nose are inserted for a few minutes gauze sponges soaked with rosehip oil, and then this procedure is repeated up to 5 times a day.

In nursing mothers rosehip oil will help with the problem of cracked nipples.

In addition to a pronounced healing effect on the body, rosehip oil is an effective anti-depressant. Include it in your daily diet to combat neurological disorders, for getting rid of uncertainty in your own abilities and in general to raise the mental attitude.

Rosehip oil is sold in pharmacies. Sometimes it is sold in the form of gelatin capsules with dosed amount of oil inside.

Rosehip oil in cosmetology: For the face, neck and the hair

Despite its other useful properties, rosehip oil positive effect on the skin is probably its main feature. Thanks to contained in it vitamins, trace elements and fatty acids it has a regenerating and rejuvenating effects on the skin, improves its elasticity, eliminates irritation, normalizes the secretion of sebaceous glands. With regular use of oil increases the protective properties of the epidermis, it prevents the accumulation of the enzymes and degradation products, improves the intracellular exchange. Furthermore, rosehip oil – is a natural UV filter. It is suitable for aging, dry skin and is a good anti-aging tool to help in the fight against fine lines and pigmentation spots. It will also help relieve signs of fatigue, tone the blood vessels and give the skin of the face and neck an smooth and healthy color. It is ideal for skin care around the eyes and the delicate skin around the mouth, and if desired, it can be applied on the entire face. To saturate the skin with nutrients, rosehip oil moisturize and soften it.

Oil of rose hips strongly is contraindicated to owners of oily and acne-prone skin rash, because it can provoke the emergence of new inflammation.

For facial skin care, hair and decollete, rosehip oil can be used in pure form or as part of the usual cosmetics. With it can be enriched the washing gels, shampoos, conditioners, masks, creams, lotions and other agents in proportions of 1 to 10.

Pure rosehip oil is often used as the base oil for the preparation of medicinal aromatic mixtures. Since it may be combined with essential oils of plants such as ylang-ylang, rose, orange, lavender, patchouli, bergamot, neroli and chamomile. If it used alone, it is enough three drops of oil, in evening, inflicted on the face skin to prevent premature appearance of wrinkles and to smooth out the existing ones. The oil is applied with light patting movements, not stretching the skin.

Oil of rose hips as a remedy for stretch marks

With typical regenerative properties, rosehip oil can be used for the prevention of skin stretch marks. Its use gives good results to solve this problem as when used alone, and in combination with essential oils of rosemary, neroli and petitgrain.

Essential oils for sleeping (insomnia). Massage, oil burner and internal use of essential oils to sleep.

Before proceeding to the description of the essential oils that can help with insomnia, you need to understand the causes of this condition. Insomnia - this is a problem with falling asleep or early awakening, or a complete lack of sleep. Experts say that these symptoms may be caused by increased anxiety, very strong sense of responsibility and internal unconscious fears. Therefore, you should pay attention to your reactions, to the harmony of contacts with the outside world. If a person is constantly tense, afraid of something and feels a sense of guilt, insomnia is free to appear. After all that we have so carefully hide during the day, fully manifested at night. Therefore, to treat insomnia essential oils are simply irrational. They help to relax and put in order the nerves with minor or temporary sleep disorders. In chronic insomnia are powerless most powerful drugs because they do not clear the cause of illness. Of course, the drugs are euthanized artificially, but whether to or not to swallow tablets?, if is easier to remove the root cause?

Among the tips to overcome insomnia, you can find recommendations for a walk in the fresh air before going to bed, take a warm foot bath and listen to relaxing music. If this does not help, try to use essential oils. Generally, in the field of Ayurveda, experts argue that these funds should be familiar, because the strength of their influence on the body can not be compared to anything. It is a natural remedy that does not bring harm. Of course, if you are not allergic to smells and individual contraindications.

Essential oils for sleep

Please understand, here are indicated some essential oil and for which they are suitable to apply,and how to apply them correctly:

1. for those who do not sleep - oil of orange, cedar, mandarin, juniper, myrrh and cypress;
2. for those who has restless sleep – oil of lavender, neroli, chamomile and myrrh;
3. for complete relaxation - vanilla oil.

Use oil for insomnia in several ways: for massage, baths, aromatherapy and as an internal tool.

Massage with essential oils for sleep

Massage can be done in the evening or even at night, if you have a habit of waking up. At the same time, I advise to do self-massage of the ear with any selected oil. Do it with the tip of your little finger, gently massaging the inner surface of the ear. You can also massage the soles of the feet, whiskey or dig a drop of pure essential oil in your ears before going to bed and gently massage the tragus for 1-2 minutes. Rub gently the foots, because there are a lot of biologically active points, and if they are activated - instead of falling asleep you will have a feeling of cheerfulness and high tide forces. Some people do self-massage of neck and shoulder area. It is important to understand how massage can help you, and understand that this can only help empirically.

One tip: do massage at least a few days in a row, to understand its effectiveness.

Massage oil is prepared as follows: for the warp, take olive, sesame oil or corn oil, and add a few drops of any essential oil or more oils to taste. The oil is added slowly, stirred thoroughly and kept in a tightly closed vial. Bases should be added in proportion of 10 ml, and the essential oil can be taken in such proportions:

Recipe 1: geranium - 2 drops, patchouli - 3 drops, chamomile - 4 drops;

Recipe 2: lavender - 2 drops, myrrh - 1 drop, juniper - 3 drops;

Recipe 3: chamomile - 3 drops, lavender - 2 drops;

Recipe 4: rosemary – 1 drop, ginger - 3 drops.

Recipe 5: basil - 1 drop, lavender - 2 drops, orange - 1 drop.

If it is possible to make a back massage, it is better to do it with oil of lavender, juniper, rose, or valerian. Valid for this are 4th and 5th recipies with a base of sesame oil. In mental overexcitation (when thoughts swirling in your head, although the body is tired) can be carried out foot massage with pine or rosemary oils.

Aroma with essential oils for insomnia

For aromatherapy treatments use the above oil, just pour them in aroma lamp or in the locket and place beside the bed. You can also add a few drops on the pillow, if there is no special equipment. In winter, drip oil on a piece of wet cloth and put it on the battery, so that during sleep the oil gradually evaporates. The bedroom will be filled with flavor that will bring relief and peaceful sleep. You can simply drop the oil on a handkerchief and inhale deeply the pleasant scent by mixing at least two oils. For example, chamomile and ylang-ylang, chamomile and lavender.

Take into account that if you do not fall asleep and the cause is anger, the best to help will be the flavor of peppermint, jasmine or rose. It is also possible to use a composition of cedar, sandalwood, bergamot, rose, or recipe 5, adding to it the basil oil.

Sometimes, insomnia is caused by nightmares - a man wakes up from a bad dream and then a long time can not sleep. Valerian oil in combination with rose and lemon balm will help you to get rid of nightmares or lemon balm with petit grain and neroli or lemon balm and dill, lavender and rose. Saturating the air with these aromas you can help yourself to sleep.

For fast sleep helps aromatic pillow with this recipe: drip onto the pillow a drop of cedar oil, rose and lavender or put next to the bed scarf with these smells. For the same purpose suit lavender (2 drops), ylang-ylang, orange and chamomile - 1 drop. Before going to bed, try to make a few very deep breaths.

Internal use of essential oils for sleep

Internal use of essential oils can also help overcome insomnia. Take a piece of sugar, drip on him 3-5 drops of lavender and resorb it in the mouth.

Baths with essential oils for sleep

Lovers of baths can also find a remedy for insomnia. Bath itself is relaxing, and if you drip 3 drops of lavender oil, ylang-ylang and chamomile, you will fall asleep quickly, and your sleep will be strong. Baths very well help with fatigue and chronic fatigue. For those who wake up from any rustle, benzoin will be useful - an essential oil, which is made of resin from storax tree. It will help make sleep less sensitive.

Contraindications to the use of essential oils for a dream

Despite the fact that essential oil - means seem completely natural and harmless, they still contain the concentrated power plants that affect different people differently. Therefore, there is a category of people and the types of occupations in which essential oils should be used with caution. Carefully use oils in pregnant women (especially in the first half), not all oils can be given to children, people with high blood pressure, with reduced pressure, diabetes and cancer, asthma and epilepsy.

Contraindications are also a professional activity associated with high concentration of attention and responsibility for the lives of other people (driver, pilot, etc.). However, it is more correct to the use oils in the daytime.

Essential oil of nutmeg: composition and properties. Muscat oil in cosmetics, cooking and aromatherapy.

Among the wonders of Mother Nature's essential oils can be called one of the most amazing. It really a terrific gift: tiny drops of oil that people have learned to isolate from plants for thousands of years ago, these drops contain many useful, and have such powerful healing properties, which no one drug have. Besides essential oils are safe when we properly handle with them.

Muscat oil, like many essential oils, has rich composition and is used in many areas: for the diseases treatment, rehabilitation, wellness and health, as well as in cooking - the aroma of this oil is called "warming".

Nutmeg grows in the equatorial belt; is an evergreen tree, reaching 20 meters in height. Already the tree itself is surprising: it begins to blossom after 5-6 years, and does not cease to bloom all his life - and the life of nutmeg can be long - up to 100 years. About 40 of them tree bearing fruits - from 3 to 10 thousand nuts per year. These nuts resemble in appearance a peach, but in the size they are smaller; essential oil extracted from the nutmeg seed and shell of the nut – is called oil of mace, but it is rarely used today.

It is believed that nutmeg comes from the islands in the Western Pacific - such as the Moluccas; grow it mainly in Indonesia, Sri Lanka, in India, in Africa and in Grenada - one of the islands of the Caribbean. Muscat oil was used in ancient times less than the oil of mace, but it also has a rich history. Egyptians - famous surgeons and embalmers used it in funeral rites - it perfectly preserved mummy; Hindus used in disorders of the stomach and intestines; inhabitants of the Roman Empire fumigated the room with it, and it was used in a mixture with other oils to protect themselves from the plague. Later, in the Middle Ages, nutmeg oil began to be used more for the treatment of hemorrhoids - from which is prepared the ointment on the basis of pork fat. Then, nutmeg and oil out of it began to be used in cooking, perfumes and cosmetics, the production of alcoholic beverages.

Composition and healing properties of nutmeg oil

The composition of nutmeg oils is complex - natural hydrocarbons and alcohols, oil derivatives which give the peculiar smell and affect its therapeutic properties. The smell of nutmeg oil is quite hot and spicy, and it can improve the perception and calm in excessive excitation.

Muscat oil has a number of therapeutic actions: analgesic, anti-inflammatory, antioxidant, anti-emetic, antiseptic, antibacterial, anti-rheumatic, healing and astringent. It eliminates pain and inflammation, reduces swelling, so it is used in neuralgia, neuritis, osteochondrosis, myositis, arthritis, muscle pain, gout, bacterial infections.

Oil cleans bronchi and increases the elasticity of the walls; It helps with uterine bleeding and nasal bleeding; can stop the blood in hemorrhages.

On the reproductive system of men and women, it has a tonic effect, and can work like estrogen - the female sex hormone. As a result, its decreases recurrent pain in women, normalize menstruation, dysfunctional disorders disappear during menopause. In addition, nutmeg oil is considered to be an effective aphrodisiac - it is prescribed for the treatment of impotence, as an additional tool; It also helps in childbirth, increasing uterine contractions.

Muscat oil in case of problems with digestion
Very effective is the oil of nutmeg in digestive problems: it contributes to better digestion of food - greasy and starchy, and improves appetite; relieves nausea, it helps with chronic diarrhea and vomiting, prevents constipation and removes bad breath. It has an antibacterial effect, so it is used in intestinal infections; It facilitates the treatment of gallstones.

Since the oil of nutmeg has a warming effect, it improves blood circulation and heart activity, it can be used as a natural stimulator. Before extracting from nutmeg the essential oil, from it is removed all fatty oils - a total weight of about 25-40% nuts. Fatty oil from nutmeg has an orange-red color, and smells good.

From purified nuts and from the husk throw steam distillation process, a volatile oil is obtained. The composition of nutmeg oil, obtained in different regions is not very different, but the oil from the western regions of India does not have the spicy smell, then other oils: its flavor seems rougher, because there are a lot of terpenes.

Muscat oil in cooking
In cooking, nutmeg oil is used as a refined seasoning - Many cooks like its sweet-tart, spicy and warm aroma.

The usual dinner can please with novelty, and even create an atmosphere of mystery, if you add a little nutmeg oil in dishes - a few drops. For example, in meat dishes and salads you can add just 1-2 drops. In the dough for baking or creams for cakes, too, do not add more than 2 drops - at the rate per kilogram of finished product.You can mix the oil of nutmeg with jam or honey, and with this mixture lubricate biscuits and buns; butter flavored wines, liqueurs and other alcoholic drinks, coffee and tea.

Muscat oil in cosmetics

In cosmetology nutmeg oil is not used as often as it can irritate the skin. However, it can be very useful if used in small doses: it rejuvenates the skin, stimulates cell regeneration, improves circulation. If you rub a mixture of oils with the addition of nutmeg into the scalp, it improves hair growth, and they will become stronger.

Externally the oil is used for muscular and rheumatic pains – in 10 ml of base add 5-10 drops; in creams, shampoos, tonics and shower gels - 4 drops of oil on conventional disposable portion.

Internal just one drop, adding it to a cup of tea with herbs: overexciting, poor appetite, flatulence, diarrhea, intestinal infections, manifestations of menopause and menstrual irregularities.

Nutmeg oil in aromatherapy

In aromatic lamp pour 5-7 drops of nutmeg oil; for making oil bath (1-10 drops) are dissolved in milk (2 tablespoons) and then poured into water.

With nutmeg oil impose you may do massage: in 10 ml of base - 5-10 drops.

During epidemics of influenza and SARS oil can be flavored indoor: it destroys viruses, cleans the air and stimulates the immune system.

Fragrance of oil helps to relieve stress, to feel at ease in a difficult situation - for example, before public speaking, or during the holiday organization - it gives vivacity and energy.

With the help of nutmeg oil can be easier to get a new team, learn a new activity and learn to not be afraid to take responsibility.

Contraindications

Contraindications to the use the nutmeg oil are: increased nervous irritability, mental disorders, epilepsy, pregnancy, age < 18 years.

It is believed that the essential oil of nutmeg because of the presence of myristicin and safrole can be poisonous. Myristicin - a psychoactive drug that can cause hallucinations, and safrole also can have a narcotic effect, so oil overdose is unacceptable.

Oil of nutmeg may be combined with many other essential oils like: patchouli, geranium, mandarin, juniper, tea tree, rosemary, black pepper, cinnamon, coriander, clove, cypress, sandalwood, etc.

Nutmeg oil must be store in a cool, dark place in a tightly sealed container - so it can be stored for about 2 years.

Apricot kernel oil: structure, properties and applications. Apricot kernel oil in cosmetics for the face, hair and nails.

Apricot kernel oil is obtained by cold pressing of apricot pits. In some cases, the production of oil is mixed with plum cores.

The composition of apricot kernel oil

Apricot kernel oil is classified as basic (fatty) oil. It has a light yellow transparent color and has a bland flavor. The consistency of oil is slightly viscous liquid. The composition of apricot kernel oil is similar to the peach and almond oils, also relating to base.

Such oils are often used undiluted or used as a basis for various oil mixtures. The apricot kernel oil contains a lot of vitamins, minerals (potassium, magnesium), mono- and polyunsaturated fatty acids (palmitic, stearic, linoleic, linolenic, etc.). In particular vitamin A, which promotes natural hydration of the skin and retains its elasticity, vitamin C, which provides the elasticity of the skin and the F vitamin, normalizes the sebaceous glands and accelerates skin regeneration.

Apricot kernel oil: properties, application, treatment

Apricot kernel oil has anti-inflammatory, regenerating and toning effect. It is suitable for all skin types, including delicate skin of babies and the skin exposed to age-related changes. It can help you get rid of prickly heat, diaper rash, and seborrheic dermatitis in infants, to accelerate the healing of wounds and bruises, to get rid of cellulite, soften the hardened skin and smooth out wrinkles. Apricot kernel oil is a good moisturizer and gives the skin a beautiful flat, and most importantly a healthy color. It has a beneficial effect both on problem skin, eliminating inflammation and dry it perfectly. Apricot kernel oil also has a number of medicinal properties, in particular, it can be used as an adjunct in the treatment of diseases of the central nervous, cardiovascular and immune system.

In addition, apricot kernel oil is widely used in the perfume and cosmetics industry as a base for creams, balms and lipsticks.

Apricot kernel oil in cosmetics.For hair, nails and skin

As mentioned above, apricot kernel oil - it is the best escape for skin lacking of vitamins, suffering from lack of hydration and proper nutrition. The range of its application to improve the condition of the skin is quite wide. According to the results of the research, apricot kernel oil:

1. softens and moisturizes the skin;
2. prevents dryness and flaking;
3. accelerates the process of exfoliation of dead cells of the epidermis;
4. tones the skin;
5. produces anti-aging effect;
6. evens the complexion;
7. removes skin inflammation.

In addition, included in the apricot kernel oil ingredients furthermore stimulate the synthesis of collagen and elastin, which form the basis of connective tissue of the human body.

With it you can lubricate the face before bedtime, apply a small amount on the eyelids, and the dots on the problem areas of the skin (peeling, inflammation, hardened seats). In just a heated state apricot kernel oil is effective as a cleansing lotion to remove makeup and daily cleansing of skin. Oil from apricot kernels - it is also a saving for owners of sensitive skin that reacts negatively to various cosmetics, as it soothes and it actually performs all the same functions as a conventional cream.

As for the hair and nails, the apricot oil positively influences the growth and structure, improving their condition quickly. In this regard, manufacturers of cosmetics often add it to shampoos, conditioners, liquid soaps, and other preparations. However, it is worth remembering that natural apricot kernel oil is an expensive component, and, therefore, cosmetics based on it also can not be cheap.

Recipes with apricot kernel oil

A mixture of apricot kernel oil for anti-cellulite massage: apricot kernel oil (2 tablespoons), avocado oil (2 tablespoons), essential oil of orange, lemon, rosemary and juniper (2 drops), mix well, apply on skin.

Mask with apricot kernel oil for oily skin: apricot kernel oil (1 tablespoon), essential oil of lavender, lemon and tea tree (1 drop). It can be applied in the form of applications, and entirely on the entire face, avoiding the eye area.

Mask with apricot kernel oil to relieve signs of fatigue: apricot oil (1 tablespoon), essential oil of patchouli, chamomile (1 drop).

Moisturizing formula for body: apricot kernel oil (2 tablespoons), almond oil (2 tablespoons), essential oil of ylang-ylang, sandalwood and lavender (2 drops). Apply on the body after water bath, suitable for everyday use.

Face mask for mixed type of skin: apricot kernel oil (1 tablespoon), peach oil (1 tablespoon), essential oil of ylang-ylang, lemon, neroli and mint (1 drop). Gives the skin freshness, it makes the skin uniform.

Mix for hand care and nail care: apricot kernel oil (1 tablespoon), wheat germ oil (1 tablespoon), jojoba oil (1 tablespoon). Such a mixture can be prepared in large quantities by placing it in a clean opaque jar and store in a cool place.

Enriched lotion with apricot kernel oil to cleanse the skin: apricot kernel oil (1 tablespoon), castor oil (1 tablespoon),vitamin E oil (10 drops). Ideal for dry skin.

Nourishing cream with apricot kernel oil for eyelids: apricot oil (1 tablespoon), olive oil (1 tablespoon), vitamin A in oil (1 capsule), rosehip oil (0.5 tablespoon). Apply a small amount on the eyelid skin at bedtime.

A mixture of apricot kernel oil for wrinkles: apricot oil (1 tablespoon), avocado oil (1 tablespoon), jojoba oil (1 tablespoon), rosewood essential oil (4 drops), frankincense essential oil (3 drops). It can be applied both at night and during the day on clean skin.

Natural apricot kernel oil: it is eco-friendly and non-toxic drug that can be used as in pregnant women and nursing mothers.

Peach oil: chemical composition and properties of peach oil. The use of peach oil. Mask with peach oil for the skin and eyelashes.

Oil with tenderest name "peach" is produced from seeds of peach throw mechanical pressing. The output is a light in consistency and nutritious oil, which became very popular in the pharmaceutical and cosmetics industry. In folk medicine, peach oil is also used for medicinal and cosmetic purposes.

The chemical composition of peach oil

Peach oil contains large amounts of polyunsaturated fatty acids, which are essential for the life of our skin. With palmitic, oleic, linoleic and gamma-linolenic acid, we can significantly improve the condition of skin cells. It is also unique as a part of peach oil-vitamin B15, which is beneficial and very effective for skin fading .

Separately, I can say about vitamin E, which has antioxidant and preservative properties, as well as vitamin A, which maintains the integrity of skin cells. All this testifies the rejuvenating and stopping the aging properties of peach oil. The composition of peach seed oil includes and vitamins A and P (30 to 40%), vitamin C and group B vitamins. There are also carotenoids (it coloring the fruit); tocopherols and phospholipids. From the minerals, oil have: potassium, calcium, phosphorus and iron.

The properties of peach butter

Peach oil can literally 'animate' the skin - in fact it act in a complex, immediately nourishes, moisturizes and restores it. The oil helps to prevent cell dehydration, smooths wrinkles and shallow, effectively maintains firmness and elasticity of all skin types. Especially recommend this oil for use on sensitive and inflamed skin. Long-term and systematic use of oil peach significantly strengthened vessels of the skin (the color becomes more even), and cleaned the skin pores. Dry skin is more healthy, but sensitive - more inaccessible the exposure. Skin as it tightens, it becomes a more youthful and supple.

Peach oil is also suitable for the skin around the eyes, for eyelashs and lip skin and hair care. However, over time we will open new properties of this oil, and now we will move on to the practice.

Contraindications for peach oil

Peach oil is not suitable for people with intolerance to the individual components of peach oil. Oil can be mixed with other vegetable oils to obtain a product with extended spectrum of activity or can be used alone. It is often used as a base for various cosmetic procedures, because it is great absorbed into the skin.

Dry, sensitive skin will respond gratefully to use of peach oil as a night cream and if there are affected, scaly or inflamed patches of skin - you need to apply this oil several times a day.

- You can "enrich" the cream with peach oil by adding a drop of oil directly before use (separate part of the cream and mix with butter oil).

Peach oil can be used as a cleanser to remove make-up: it should be a little warm up on water bath, them soak with it a cotton pad and remove makeup from the skin, eyes and lips.

To strengthen the skin around the eyes: you need to put oil on the right place and carefully drive it into the skin with your fingertips

For eyelash, procedure is very simple: with a clean eyelash brush apply to the eyelashes the oil an hour before bedtime. Before going to bed remove remaining oil.

For lips procedure is similar: in the skin of the lips plot the oil with any materials, with hand or finger, while not drinking and not eating for an hour. If your lips were cracked badly, you can do application with strips of cotton wool soaked in peach oil.

Mask with peach butter to the face and body

1. *Nutritional and tonic for dry and normal skin.* Take a ripe peach (take 2 tablespoons of pulp), 1 tablespoon of peach oil, ¾ tablespoon from your cream. Quickly and thoroughly mix the components of the mask and immediately apply it on the face. Hold 15 minutes, wash off with water at room temperature.
2. *Soothing mask for sensitive skin.* Take 1 tablespoon of cottage cheese, 1 tablespoon of peach oil. Simply mix all ingredients and apply on face for 15 minutes. Wash off the mask with warm water.
3. Mask-Scrub for dry and prone flaking skin. You will need 1 tablespoon of almond bran and 1 tablespoon incomplete slightly warmed oil from peach seeds. Mix the components and the resulting composition is applied to damp skin. Then you need to do gently face massage for about a minute. Hold 15 minutes, wash off with warm water.

Lotion with peach butter

1. Lotion from peach oil to cleanse dry and aging skin. You will need about 2 cups of fresh rose petals (petals of rosehip). Pour them into a separate bowl (which can be heated), fill it with peach oil, so that the petals were completely covered. Put the dish in a water bath and heat to the point where the petals lose their color completely. Then pour the liquid into a glass jar, tightly cover with a lid and leave for one day. Then strain through a strainer - now obtained lotion can be used for daily cleansing of skin.

2. Masks for eyelashes. You need finely chopped parsley, peach oil and aloe vera juice. Mix everything and add a little olive oil. Mix well until smooth. Make a layer from sterile material , put inside the mask and put it on the lash region. If you do this procedure every day for two weeks - the result will be stunning. Mask length time - 15 minutes.

   - A little bit warm peach oil, soak cotton pads with it or pieces of cotton, and then impose them on the lashes. Then cover your eyes with compress strips of paper and close the face with warm cloth. After 15 minutes, you can clean and remove oil residues.

   - Mix the peach oil with castor oil in equal proportions, or arbitrarily, and lubricate them every day eyelashes. Preferably, of course, doing it in the morning and evening. The tool is good because it is absolutely hypoallergenic.

Mask with peach butter to the hair

1. Hair Mask. You will need 2 tablespoons of peach oil, 3-5 drops of any essential oil. Both components are mixed until uniform and the resulting mixture is rubbed into the scalp, leaving 15-30 minutes. This is especially good mask for troubled, dry and brittle hair.

Essential oil of citronella: composition and properties of citronella oil. Use of citronella oil.

Citronella - it is a grass, that have a height of one meter and possesses a pronounced lemon flavor. In the wild it grows only on the island of Sri Lanka (formerly Ceylon), but is cultivated in many other Asian countries, notably in Indonesia (Java Island),

Malaysia, China, Burma and Madagascar. Citronella essential oil is obtained by steam distillation from already dried herb. Freshly picked stems of citronella are rarely used for manufacturing, for the simple reason that it requires a much larger amount of fuel, which consequently leads to a rise in the cost of the final product. Oil yield consist about 0.5-1%, which means that for the production of 1 kg of citronella oil will require at least 200 kg of raw material. It is believed that the best quality oil is produced on the Indonesian island of Java, while the historic homeland of citronella – is the island of Sri Lanka, where oil has less pronounced characteristics. The price of this kind of essential oil depends on the manufacturer and the supplier countries.

Essential oil of citronella: composition

Depending on the type of citronella grass used to prepare an essential oil, in a larger or smaller number contains components such as aldehydes - citral and citronellal, terpene alcohols - borneol, geraniol, nerol and citronellol and terpenes - camphene, dipentene and limonene.

Citral, acting as flavoring agent, is used in perfumery and food industries. It is part of the ocular drugs and has properties of lowering blood pressure. In addition, the citral is a raw material for synthesizing vitamin A. The terpene alcohols often act as components of perfume compositions and is used in the manufacture of soaps and household products, and terpenes - are generally a leading component of resins and balsams. They are also used in the production of fragrances and perfumes as in the perfume and cosmetic industries.

Properties and application of essential oils of citronella

Citronella oil, unlike most other essential oils has a rather limited list of useful properties. Moreover, its main advantage - *the ability to scare away all kinds of insects.* For this reason, at the time, add citronella oil in your candle wax, so as to not only illuminate the room, but at the same time scare away mosquitoes. A drop of essential oil of citronella added in sachets for wardrobe will not only give *a fresh scent* to your laundry, but will not allow *moths.* The oil diluted with water and atomized by spraying, protect your home from *pesky insects, freshen the air, and even neutralizes tobacco smoke, and added to the dishwashing liquid, it eliminates unpleasant smells (grease, fish, onions, garlic).*

The therapeutic properties of essential oil of citronella are similar to the properties of essential oil of other herb – like palmarosa, in connection with which they can be interchanged. Oil of citronella is considered a *good antiseptic* and is recommended for *skin inflammations.* It is used in *vegetative-vascular dystonia, regular bouts of weakness, dizziness, disorders of the vestibular apparatus.* Citronella oil has a

72

stimulating effect on the *human immune system* and enhance health in general. It is used as an aid for the period of rehabilitation after complicated operations and strong injuries, as well as during physical exertion. According to some data can improve the *sharpness of hearing, and get rid of extraneous noise in the ears.* The most positive effects of essential oil of citronella is it effect on the *digestive tract, improving the process of digestion and eliminate the possibility of an enzyme deficiency. It also helps to remove toxins from the body and inhibits excessive appetite.*

Contraindications for citronella oil

Citronella oil is contraindicated for pregnant women, in high blood pressure, and people who are prone to rapid overexcitement. It can not be used inside with high acidity, gastric ulcer, gastritis and can not be applied to sensitive and prone to irritation skin. In industry citronella essential oil is used in the manufacture of perfumes, deodorants, soaps, various cosmetics and household chemical products.

Influence of citronella oil on the psycho-emotional state

Citronella oil - is *the oil of joy, vigor and vitality.* Inhale its aroma and you can feel the surge of energy and feel a strong emotional outburst. It awakens the desire to communicate and can even coerce any adventure. Citronella essential oil relieves depression and indifference to reality, prompting the man to move forward to the unknown. In addition, it is known, *it can improve concentration, increase memory capacity and enhance the ability to quickly assimilate information.*

Given the above and the fact that citronella has *tonic properties,* this oil can be recommended for drivers of cars and other vehicles. It is also believed that the essential oil of citronella – it is an aphrodisiac that can *enhance the potency* and awaken sexual activity, both women and men.

Essential oil of citronella: methods of application

With citronella oil may *be enriched cosmetics* by adding 3-4 drops in 15 g. of the base, adding *in your massage cream* - 5 drops to 20 ml of base, *into the bath or immediately before its adoption* - 10 drops to the bath. To carry out the procedures of aromatherapy with citronella, add 5-6 drops of essential oil into aroma lamp, its enough for the area up *to 15 sq.m.* When oil is ingested (1 drop at a time), it is necessarily to be mixed with honey or jam, dripping on the dried fruit or a slice of bread crumb. At the same time it should be abundantly drink with warm tea, with water or yogurt.

By combining citronella with other oils, remember that the best results can be achieved by combining it with essential oils of *bergamot, ylang-ylang, lavender, peppermint, sage and eucalyptus.*

Chamomile essential oil: composition, useful properties and applications of chamomile oil. Chamomile oil for hair use, cosmetics, skin and nails.

Chamomile essential oil - the result of a steam distillation of its inflorescences. To produce 1 kg of oil is required at least 200 kg of raw material. Thus, it is necessary to distinguish between types of chamomile used for the production of essential oils.

The most "young" oil made from chamomile Moroccan (Ormenis multicaulis), which grows as the name implies, in the northwest of Africa. It is also grown in the south of Spain and in Israel. Oil appeared on the market relatively recently and therefore is not very popular.

The most expensive raw material for essential oil is considered to be Roman chamomile (Anthemis nobilis). It looks like a wild chrysanthemum and grow in European countries with temperate climates, especially in Belgium, France, Hungary, Germany and the UK. Moreover, a few decades ago, the main producer of this oil was England, in connection with which the trade name was used frequently: English Daisy (Camomile English).

Finally, the most common essential oils are made from blue or German chamomile, which, in fact, is the same. This type (Matricaria chamomilla, Chamomilla recutita) grows everywhere in Russia, Europe, western Asia, and is cultivated in Australia and North America. The price of chamomile oil ranges from 3 dollars per 10 ml.

The composition of the essential oil of chamomile

Chamomile oil usually has a blue color. However, depending on the temperature and the storage time, the color can change from green to brown. Have a thick consistency, herbal aroma of tart with a hint of tobacco, hay and sweet spices. On the chemical composition significantly affects the time of collection of raw material and the stage of plant development. The essential oil of chamomile in sufficient quantity contained substances such as hamazulen and bisabolol, which are often used in the manufacture of infant and hypoallergenic cosmetics, products for tanning, aftershaves and perfumes. Both substances have an effective sedative, anti-inflammatory and soothing effect. Products are rather expensive, so their synthetic analogues are frequently used in the industry.

In addition, the composition of chamomile oil include various hydrocarbon compounds - farnesene, kadin, terpinenes and so on.

Chamomile essential oil: useful properties, application

The beneficial properties of chamomile essential oil has been known for several thousand years ago. For centuries, starting from the time of ancient Egypt, chamomile was used as a powerful antiseptic, and the ancient Greek physician Hippocrates, with it help the people to treat the malaria.

Chamomile essential oil has *antibacterial, anti-inflammatory, tonic, analgesic and wound-healing properties.* This detrimental effect on the number of pathogenic bacteria make oil effectively in use as an aid in diseases such as *angina, bronchitis, laryngitis, pneumonia and conjunctivitis (daisy water).* Its use and other respiratory diseases, as it can reduce body temperature when feverish.

Chamomile oil *enhances the immune system, stimulates appetite and has a positive effect on the function of the gastrointestinal tract, including stomach ulcers and duodenal ulcers.* It is also believed that it is useful for women's health in disorder of the menstrual cycle and during menopause.

In general, the properties of chamomile oil is similar to the properties of lavender oil, with the only difference being that the essential oil of lavender is recommended in the presence of acute pain, and chamomile essential oil - for chronic pain. Useful in the emotional sphere, using chamomile essential oil the irritability can be removed, unfounded fears and excessive excitement. It helps to cope with insomnia, relieves tension and stabilizes emotions. In addition, chamomile oil has a positive effect on the work of the brain and activates the memory. *Use 2 drops of oil per teaspoon of honey inside, twice, daily.*

Contraindications

Chamomile essential oil is contraindicated in pregnant women and children under the age of six years. It is also not recommended to combine with the use of homeopathic medicines, since it cancels its revitalizing effect.

The use of chamomile essential oil in cosmetics, for hair, skin and nails

Chamomile essential oil has a fairly diverse cosmetic effect. First of all, it well *relieves inflammation in the sun and thermal burns, insect bites.* It helps in healing wounds and open sores. Secondly, it is often used for treatment of *alopecia* induced by various causes. Regular use of chamomile oil for hair, *stimulates their growth, nourishes and restores the structure.* Over time, hair becomes shiny, silky and more durable. It is also believed that the essential chamomile oil (blue) removes dandruff and even hair lightens. Third, chamomile oil is indispensable for the *care of dry, sensitive and prone to irritation skin.* It easily reduces inflammation, itching, relieves acne, blackheads and pustular rash, whitens the skin of the face and hands, smoothes fine lines. Long-term use of oil can solve the problem *of broken vessels (rosacea) and to eliminate allergic reactions.*

It is useful as a preventive agent for *the narrowing of blood vessels and maintain the natural, healthy complexion.* And finally, fourthly, chamomile oil is recommended for infections caused by ingrown nails, for faster cuticle healing. With chamomile oil can be enriched cosmetics (creams, gels, toners, masks for the face, body and hair) .Add 3 drops to 5 grams bases; with oil aromatize bath (8-10 drops), add for the massage cream (7 drops to 10 ml of base oil).

To achieve different results Chamomile essential oil blends well with oils such as bergamot, bigard (bitter orange), geranium, cypress, lavender, petitgrain, rose and rosewood.

Stone oil: chemical composition, the use and contraindications. stone oil treatment. Crack stone oil.

It is a liquid that oozes out of rocks and hardens with time in the air. Stone oil is also called mountain wax or white stone of immortality. The hunters watched the animals licking stones and could not understand why they do it. At a closer look, they saw that it was not just the stones, but the hardened resin stone. It is a real wealth, because the stone oil contains minerals, trace elements able to establish balance in the body and normalize blood chemistry.

This is very important in oncology, when the body does not have enough strength to deal with infringement in the cellular metabolism. However, the stone oil can be used virtually in all diseases because it effectively contributes to the protective functions of the organism. Thus, the application of this oil is very rapid regeneration of skin, bone and mucosa.

The chemical composition of the stone oil

Stone oil belongs to the group of alum. It contains a large amount of iron, copper, zinc, manganese, selenium, nickel, chromium, vanadium, cobalt, titanium. There are also other trace elements, which normalize the blood homeostasis.

The mechanism of action of stone of immortality is that when it is used, each cell of a body has the ability to take away from him so many trace elements, as it is required for a full existence.

This version of the official medicine, which took the stone oil on board. A traditional healers also speak of the strong funds power, and call it "tears of the mountains". Stones have been so much time in their development, that they have absorbed as much solar energy and soaked natural vibrations of the earth, that their tears carry all the power and force of nature, part of which is the man. The particles of nature, enclosed in a stone oil, adjust the human body, like a tuning fork, on natural vibrations - vibrations that carry harmony and health.

Contraindications to the use of stone oil

Stone oil is contraindicated in obstructive jaundice, because it reveals a very strong choleretic effect.

Also, do not take the stone oil for constipation, because toxins outputted drug from the body. In this case, you must first provide a daily stool with a special diet, fermented milk products, or enemas, and then use medicines on the basis of stone oil.

Caution: during the reception of funds from the oil stone is better not to drink black tea, coffee, cocoa, chocolate, because teeth can turn yellow. You also can not take alcohol, antibiotics, meat: duck, goose, pork and lamb, as well as radish.

Stone oil treatment: application

In what diseases used stone oil:

    a. Gastric ulcer;
    b. Tuberculosis;
    c. Hemorrhoids;

d. Poisoning;

e. Frostbite;

f. Myoma;

g. Streptoderma;

h. Diseases of the liver and kidneys;

i. Erosion;

j. Gynecological disorders;

k. Tumors;

l. Diseases of the oral cavity;

m. Stroke;

n. Epilepsy;

This list can be continued, because there is no such condition in which the stone oil would have been powerless.

Cure from stone oil

This tool really is a kind of pebbles of different colors - from yellow to brown, sometimes with a reddish tinge. You need to crush the stones into powder and the powder must be dissolved in water. At 0.5 liters of water (raw or boiled), you need to add 2.5 grams of hard powder. Take 1 tablespoon up to three times a day before meals. The resulting yellow precipitate must be drained and use as an external agent.

The cure in this way should be from 5 to 7 days, then make a three-day (sometimes one-day) break, then do another course.

Despite the fact that oil is not a stone mined on an industrial scale, it is advantageous in fact that for the treatment should be used a very small amount. For example, 5 grams of hard butter are enough for a course of treatment. Even for a cure for stomach ulcers or tuberculosis you only need 10g of powder - tested in practice.

Application for the treatment of stone oil

Stone oil for prostatitis.

In this disease are used microclysters. In 0.5 liters of boiled water dissolve 3 g of hard butter. Then, clean the intestines and immediately make microclysters with volume of 30-40 ml, better warm. The course of treatment - 1 month.

Stone oil for hemorrhoids.

In 600 ml of warm water dissolve 3g. of stone powder. Do microclysters in amount of 30-40 ml daily. The course of treatment last - 2 weeks. If the problem persists, extend for a further 2 weeks.

Stone oil for uterine myoma and erosion.

- In 1 liter of boiled water dissolve 3 g of stone powder. Drink 1 glass 3 times a day for half an hour before a meal, but if there are problems with acidity - better to drink hour before.
- You can also use tampons. For this purpose in 0.5 liters of boiled water dissolve 3 g of hard butter. Moisten the swab tool and carefully insert into the vagina, keep on all night long.

Stone oil against deposition of salts.

In 2 liters of boiled water dissolve 3 g of hard butter. Take a glass 3 times a day for half an hour before meals. In increased acidity - take at least one hour before a meal. In this case, the treatment is quite long - from 3 months to a year.

Treatment for stomach ulcers with stone oil.

In 600 ml of boiling water dissolve 3 g of stone powder. Take 1 tablespoon 3 times a day for half an hour before meals.

Stomach cancer.

The recipe is the same as in ulcer, but the course of treatment will last from 3 months to a year.

Stone oil for diabetes.

For a full course you need 72 g.. It will last about 80 days. In 2 liters of water dissolve 3 g of stone powder and take for 80 days. Thus, it is necessary to monitor the level of sugar, and do every week your sugar analysis. Do not impair the physician prescribing. After one month of the course make a break and then repeat the course.

Stone oil for sinusitis.

First, do a warm bath, then a lotion from stone oil. The solution is prepared as follows: 3 g of stone powder in 300 ml of boiled water. Wetting the gauze in the lotion and impose it in the nose. The procedure is carried out in a day. The course of treatment - 12 days/ 1 procedure per day.

Treatment for wounds and burns.

Prepare disinfectant solution: in 300 ml of water, add 3 g of hard butter, use this tool as iodine.

Stone oil for colon cancer.

In 500 ml of boiled water dissolve 3 g of stone powder. Drink 1 glass 3 times a day for half an hour before meals, in high acidity take at least an hour before. In one day you will require 4,5 g. of powder, take the cure 3 or 4 months. At the same time make a clear solution for microclysters by scheme: 3 grams of stone powder diluted in 600 ml of boiled water, add 2 tbsp. of honey. The circuit is a uniform distribution of time between enemas. In the treatment of cancer, it is desirable at the same time with the treatment with stone oil to take special anti-inflamatory herbs.

Do not violate drug regimen prescribed by your doctor.

Anise oil: composition. Useful properties and treatment with essential oil of anise. The use of anise oil in cosmetics for the face, body and hair.

Essential oil of anise (anise oil) - product of distillation of the ordinary anise seeds, annual plant which grows in South and North America, some African countries, India, and southern Europe. A plant that grows in culture up to 60 cm in height, has a small white flowers and gray-brown seeds.

Anise oil: composition

To produce 1 kg of essential oil of anise requires about 50 kg of mature seeds, which are first crushed, and only then subjected to a process of distillation. By reducing the temperature of the oil, it becomes a dense structure and freezes, so it is recommended to warm before using it for a while in the hands.

The main component of anise oil – is anethole, 80-90% of all matter. Another important component - methyl chavicol, organic matter phenol series, the content of which in the essential oil of anise is 10%. Furthermore, this type of oil includes: a-phellandrene, a-pinene, acetaldehyde anisketon, dipentene and camphene.

Anise oil is classified as hard drug, so it is not advised to use in pregnant women, and people with very sensitive skin, to avoid possible skin irritation.

Essential oil of anise: useful properties, treatment

Anise oil has a wide range of therapeutic and preventive effects. Firstly, it is effective for colds, in particular affecting the respiratory system as an expectorant and has a soothing effect and is also a febrifuge. And thanks to a warming property as a whole will improve the general condition at colds of varying severity. Secondly, anise essential oil improves the digestive tract, stimulates peristalsis, help in colic, flatulence and dyspepsia (early satiety, feeling of heaviness in the stomach). It also relieves nausea and vomiting caused by primarily neurological disorders. In some cases, the use of anise oil can get rid of constipation. Third, anise essential oil has anti-inflammatory effects on the urinary tract and kidney tissue. It acts as a diuretic drug and it is often prescribed as an adjunct in the treatment of such diseases as oliguria (decreased urine output).

In addition, anise oil is effective for problems of a sexual nature, namely, impotence in men and frigidity in women. About these properties of anise even know the inhabitants of ancient Rome, who considered it an aphrodisiac and included it in their nutritious diet. Today it is also known that in the composition of the essential oil of anise was found the presence of the hormone estrogen, has a positive effect also on human reproduction.

Female body gratefully accept anise oil during irregular cycle, painful menstruation and long delivery process, because it can muffle the pain. In nursing mothers it can increase lactation, if necessary.

It is also believed that the essential oil of anise stimulates the appetite, relieves hangover syndrome and relieves migraines and long headache. Influence the emotional state of a person, anise oil gives the force in mental fatigue; reduces the manifestation of chronic fatigue syndrome; It calms under stress and removes from depression; It inspires human to be optimistic; It helps to cope with the states of jealousy and anger. With regard to children, in this case, anise oil is able to relieve them from excessive tearfulness and excitability. Anise oil is used primarily for the care of skin. It improves skin elasticity, normalizes water-fat balance, increases the overall tone and gives it a youthful and healthy appearance. Helps in the treatment of various skin diseases, is effective for getting rid of head lice and scabies.

Anise oil enrich the funds for hair care (shampoos, conditioners), body (gels, lotions), face (creams, tonics), it is added to mixtures for massage and aroma baths. In the enrichment of cosmetic take the proportion of 3 drops to a 10 ml. basis, for massage: 3 drops of oil per 10 g of carrier oil (or cream), for bath take 7 drops per bath.

Anise oil, in principle, like any other, especially enhanced in the bath or sauna, expanding the pores of the skin exposed to high temperatures, which contributes to more rapid penetration of nutrients of essential oil in the human body.

Mixture for massage with anise oil for skin tightening
Mixture for skin tightening after childbirth and weight loss.

Ingredients: 30 ml of base oil (apricot, jojoba, almond, hazelnut), essential oil - 3 drops of anise, petitgrain -3 drops, rosemary -3 drops. Rub into the problem areas with light massage movements after taking a bath. Surplus.

Aroma bath with anise oil.

Composition of the mixture: emulsifier (milk, cream)-100 ml, essential oils - 3 drops of anise, lemon- 3 drops, 3 drops of rosemary. Add to a filled bath with comfortable temperature, soak not more than 20 minutes there.

Anti-cellulite bath with anise oil.

The composition of the mixture: 100 g of sea salt, essential oil - 3 drops of anise, vetiver- 1 drop, grapefruit- 4 drops, peppermint- 1 drop. Oils are mixed with salt and then the resulting mixture is added to water. Bathing time- do not exceeding 30 minutes. Bath can be accompanied by a massage.

In some cases red or white wine may be used as an emulsifier.

Anise oil well fit with these types of essential oils: clove, cardamom, cedar, laurel, coriander, mandarin orange, fennel, cumin, fennel, amyris, ferrule and rosewood. The main thing to remember is the sense of proportion, and that many of the oils are potent.

Mango butter: composition, properties, application, and treatment. Essential oil of mango in cosmetics for the face, body and hair.

Mango butter is extracted from the seeds of the Indian Mangifery (Mangifera indica), better known to us as the mango. His birthplace, as we see in it names, is India, but now there are mango plantations in North, South and Central America, in several Asian countries, in the tropical belt of Africa, as well as in Australia. Mango is cultivated even in Europe, mainly in Spain and the Canary Islands. Mature fruits can reach a weight of more than two kilograms and have or one-color (green, yellow or red), or a multi-colored fruit.

Mango oil: composition

Mango oil belongs to a group of solid vegetable oils, called butter. It has a semisolid consistency at room temperature, and begins to melt at a temperature of 40 ° C. Mango oil has a neutral flavor and its color can vary from white to pale yellow or cream.

The chemical composition of mango butter is characterized primarily by monounsaturated triglycerides of the following acids: oleic, stearic, palmitic, linoleic, linolenic and arachidic. As it also contains vitamins (A, E, C, E and group B), folic acid and minerals (iron, potassium, calcium and magnesium). In addition, the oil composition comprises phytosterols and tocopherols, components that are the source of active ingredients to the epidermis.

Mango butter: properties, use and treatment

Mango butter, or as it is called by experts "mango seed oil", has a wide range of actions that are: anti-inflammatory, regenerating, moisturizing, soothing and photoprotectiv. It is recommended for treatment of certain skin diseases such as dermatitis, psoriasis, eczema and dry forms of various skin rashes. Many use it to get rid of muscle pain, relieve tension and fatigue, and therefore the mango butter is often included in the composition of mixtures for massage. In addition, it is believed that it helps in case of itching from insect bites. Mango oil restores the natural lipid barrier of the skin, restoring its ability to retain moisture, so it can be used after a sauna, bath or pool, as well as to eliminate the effects of other skin drying up of factors, such as sunburn, frostbite, chapping.

Yet the main purpose of the mango seed oil - is the daily care of the skin, hair and nails. It is equally suitable for normal and combination use, for the youth and the mature skin, dry and prone to irritation. It is also indispensable for people with sensitive and flaky skin. As a result of its use, the face and body skin become soft, velvety and moisturized throughout the day. Mango butter helps in the fight against unhealthy skin color and pigment spots. It is also effective for rough skin as it softens and smoothes. In addition, when it is used regularly, mango butter is considered a good means of preventive appearance of stretch marks.

It can even be used instead of cream and after shave, it will prevent the appearance of irritation and soothe the skin quickly.

Mango oil, due to its chemical composition, its stable to oxidation, have high viscosity and a good stability of the emulsion - a welcome ingredient in various cosmetic products. Cosmetics manufacturers include it in an amount of up to 5% in creams and lotions for the body, shampoo and hair conditioners.

It is also used to create sunscreens and means to care for skin after sunburn, as it contains a large amount of unsaponifiable fractions, providing for protection from exposure to ultraviolet rays. Mango seed oil has an effective impact on the skin of the face and body, hair and nails. It can also can enrich the conventional cosmetics, as a rule, creams (in proportion 1 to 1) or hair conditioners.

Oil from Mango for hair

For hair care mango butter in a small amount is mixed with balm for hair (in a ratio of 1 to 10). The resulting mixture is applied to the hair, evenly distribute them and easily rubb into the scalp. Then wash off with water at a comfortable temperature 5-7 minutes.

Alternatively, you can try to massage the scalp with a mixture of two oils: mango and jojoba oil, mixed in equal proportions.

Active ingredients from mango butter envelop each hair, gently stroking their scales and simultaneously nourishing, moisturizing and repairing the hair along the entire length. The result is a docile, easy to comb and shiny hair that is less broken. They not only look healthy, but they are inside established.

Mango butter for the face and body

To care the skin and body there are effective mask applications with mango butter. All areas of the body that require special care, are lubricated with natural mango butter or impose on them napkins impregnated by butter. The procedure is repeated twice a day at an acute need, and once a week as a preventative. You can alternate the use of pure oil of mango or its mixtures with essential oils, at the rate of 5 drops per 10 ml of base. You also may do pleasant bath with mango butter. A small part of butter should just throw in a warm bath and soak in it for a while. It neutralizes the hardness of water and moisturize the skin.

Mango butter can also be rubbed into the nail plate at night, or at least for a few hours without washing. With regular use, your nails will be strong and solid.

When using mango butter, it should be remembered that this butter, it is distributed poorly in the skin, while in the solid state. However, is enough to heat it up a bit, and it is easily absorbed into the skin, hair and nails, without leaving any oily sensation.

Neroli: properties and composition. Contraindications and warnings for the use of essential oil of neroli. Neroli for skin use.

Essential oils - are the nature power conductors, which harmonize the general condition of the human body. They are helpful without exception, but each has the characteristic properties that help in specific situations. That is why it important to know what kind of oil is used for what.

Our theme - the oil of neroli. This unusual name is not tied to any existing plants or trees, as we used to. According to legend, neroli essential oil is named after a native of Italy - Princess Anna Maria, Countess of Neroli. Princess loved this oil and use it instead of perfume, perfuming them their belongings and making baths scented with oil of neroli. It is a strong floral aroma fragrance, attracting the attention of men and the envy of women.

The oil of neroli is prepared from petals of orange trees, and to get 800g of neroli oil, it is necessary to collect one ton of petals. Therefore, oil is quite expensive. It turns out it by forcing steam. Is produced neroli oil in France, Italy, Morocco and Portugal. It has one of the most exquisite flavors and fragrances used in the production of the highest class.

Types of neroli oil

There are three types of essential oils of neroli:

1. First is produced from the petals of the bitter Seville orange, it is called neroli-bigareyd and is considered the best from all varieties;
2. The second is made from sweet orange petals from Portugal, called "portuguese neroli";
3. Third is produced from the flowers of lemon and mandarin, and referred to simply as "neroli".

The properties and composition of the essential oil of neroli

Neroli essential oil is considered a good tranquilizer. It has beneficial effects on the nervous system, relieving people from stress. This is an excellent remedy for insomnia, especially in depressive states. Neroli oil helps with headaches, neuralgia and dizziness. It gives a sense of tranquility.

Neroli is considered good antispasmodic as it soothes intestines, helping with colitis and diarrhea. It can be used as a carminative and digestion stimulating agent.

Neroli have good effect on the cardiovascular system: it can reduce the heart rate, stimulate blood circulation, gives the tone to the whole organism.

In the sexual sphere Neroli oil will help to remove the emotional depression, you will feel liberated, so it is considered an aphrodisiac. For those who have the critical days and feel not quite well, neroli oil will serve as a sedative and easy analgesic. Exactly the same effect it will have during menopause.

As for external means, neroli oil is considered a good antiseptic, its bactericidal effect opened the first manufacturers. Also, it perfectly softens the skin, giving it an unusually aromatic floral scent. Especially helpful is the oil for dry, sensitive and aging skin.

The composition of essential oil of Neroli
It consist from nitrogen compounds include natural alcohols, terpenes and esters.

Contraindications and warnings for the use of neroli
Neroli essential oil has a relaxing effect on the body. Therefore, in those cases when you need the reaction rate, a clear head and focus on solving the problem - it is better to keep yourself from the temptation to take advantage of this oil. Because it can act as a mild sedative. At the same time, it has a stimulant effect on the sexual sphere. In pregnancy, doctors advised to pay careful attention to the use of essential oils - Neroli oil is no exception. Its use is not recommended especially in the first 4 months of pregnancy.

Not advised to use this oil to people who are undergoing to chemotherapy for cancer.

Neroli oil for skin
In cosmetology neroli essential oil is considered one of the most effective tools that do with the skin just wonders. It obviously rejuvenates the skin, especially dry and "tired", smoothes fine wrinkles and smoothes large, helps irritated skin. Use it to remove small spider veins on the legs, threadlike veins and stretch marks, it will help to heal the cracks. Even such complex diseases as eczema, herpes and acne can be treated with the skillful use of neroli oil. The fact that it can affect the regeneration of skin cells and the rapid growth of young healthy cells.

That is why the oil of neroli is useful not only for skin, but also for hair and nails. It nourishes the cells, giving the hair elasticity and strength of nails. Its disinfectant properties help to get rid of dandruff and flaking of the scalp, from the foci of inflammation around the nails.

With self-application is necessary to take into account that neroli oil blends well with the following oils: orange, styrax, bergamot, jasmine, ylang-ylang, coriander, lavender, lime, lemon, palmarosa, pelargonium, petit-grain, rose, rosemary, sandalwood.

Application of neroli oil

a) The easiest option: drip oil on a tissue and inhale the aroma;
b) In the aromatic bulb usually pour 5-7 drops of neroli oil;
c) In simple bath (without the inclusion of other oils) add 10 drops of neroli oil;
d) Make body massage by mixing 10 ml of base oil and 5-7 drops of neroli oil;
e) Massage for the face, you can do it yourself with a few drops of neroli oil;
f) For compresses use 5-7 drops;
g) Take inside 3 drops, mixed with honey;
h) To strengthen nails: drop by drop on the nail bed, rub lightly with fingers;
i) Neroli for hair: drip 1-2 drops on a comb, comb the hair in different directions;

For the scalp and strengthen the hair you should make the composition: geranium and lavender oil - 5 drops, ylang-ylang - 1 drop, neroli oil - 2 drops, orange oil - 3 drops. Mix the ingredients together, put on the scalp, do a light massage. This procedure will not only make your hair stronger, but also help get rid of the itching and dandruff.

For restless sleep: drip 1-2 drops of oil on a damp cloth, lay beside the bed or on a radiator;

Bath for women's health. Especially useful is this bath for women after 35 years. Constituents of the composition: neroli oil - 4 drops, bergamot oil - 2 drops, peppermint oil - 2 drops, sandalwood oil - 3 drops. Mix oil, pour in the water and take a bath of up to 30 minutes at a temperature of 37-38 degrees. Bath helps to normalize the endocrine background, will enhance the sensuality and will be a superb tonic for the skin.

Geranium oil: composition, properties and treatment with geranium oil. Geranium essential oils in cosmetics, for skin, face and hair.

Essential oil of geranium (Pelargonium) - the result of steam distillation of leaves, stems and flowers from geranium plant family. The oil yield of about 1 ml. per kilogram of feedstock.

The historic birthplace of geranium is a North African country, Morocco. In Europe it was brought only in the 17th century, and it quickly spread first by its States, and subsequently began to grow even in the USA, Egypt and Japan. To date, more than 200 species of geranium were isolated, while essential for the production of geranium oil are used advantageously only two varieties: Pink or Lemon. Collection of plants takes place in the middle of summer, when appear flowering buds.

Essential oil of geranium: composition and properties

Geranium oil is extracted from the ground part of the plant that has a yellow or yellow-green color and has a specific smell of geranium with light shades of rose and mint. The chemical composition of geranium oil may vary depending on the kind of raw materials and have more than 100 components, among which particularly important are: geraniol, linalool, citronellol, nerol and terpineol.

Essential oil of geranium has a wide range of medicinal properties. First of all, it is well-known agent for the treatment of diseases "ear-nose-throat", in particular, it eliminates the pain and inflammation of the middle ear, sinuses, tonsils and pharynx, helps to relieve inflammation of the mucous membranes of the mouth and nose.

Geranium oil has the ability to remove vascular spasms, thereby relieving migraine headaches. In addition, it has a beneficial effect on the heart muscle by normalizing its work and improving microcirculation in it, eliminates the effects of ischemia and tachycardia. It is also proved that regular long-term use of geranium oil equalizes blood pressure. Essential geranium oil for topical use, it is used not less than for the internal administration. It is effective for the treatment of herpes lesions, fungal lesions of the skin, dry eczema. It can help you get rid of the parasites, like lice. As an emergency measure, geranium oil is used for pain relief and faster healing of burns of varying severity. Painkiller properties can be considered at all, "business card" of this type of oil. Dental and menstrual pain, pain in arthritis, rheumatism, various neurological diseases and hemorrhoids, cramps – is not a complete list of what is able to handle the essential oil of geranium.

While working on the emotional sphere of man, geranium oil can eliminate anxiety, get rid of the long depression, and just lift your spirits. It stimulates the nervous and mental activity, in particular, increases efficiency, reduce fatigue, give a feeling of cheerfulness and concentrates. It is recommended for older people of both sexes to improve mental and physical activity. Women over 45 can use these funds to increase its own sensuality in the process of erotic communication.

Essential oil of geranium at home

The essential oil of geranium has been used in everyday life for long time ago. Since ancient times are known properties of geranium essential oil and its protection option from flies, mosquitoes, moths, and other insects harmful to man. Moreover, it is believed that the geranium protects against witches and other evil forces, absorbs all the toxins and carcinogens, clean the air, and is a powerful stimulant of bioenergy.

Treatment with essential oil of geranium: folk recipes

When applied topically, geranium oil is combined with the so-called transport (basic) oil in different proportions. As a basis-oil may be any vegetable oil with no distinct properties.

- In treatment of burns, scars, herpes use 5 drops of geranium oil to 10 ml of carrier oil. Apply the mixture on a cotton swab and apply to the affected area several times a day. A similar proportion is suitable for cleansing the skin, eczema treatment and disposal of parasites.
- Treat hormonal diseases: 1 drop of geranium oil for the lymph nodes, which are located in the armpits. It normalizes hormonal fund by increasing the amount of estrogen in the blood.
- Treatment for headaches: 1 part of geranium oil to 3 parts of oil-base. The mixture is applied to the frontal, temporal and occipital part of the head, as well as the hands and feet.
- Treatment for otitis media: 1 part of geranium oil to 2 parts carrier oil. With the resulting mixture soak tightly twisted cotton swab and insert it into the ear canal.
- Strengthening and gums protection: 1 part of geranium oil to 4 parts base. Apply to the gums with a cotton pad.
- For mouth rinsing: geranium oil is dissolved in warm water (3 drops per 200 ml).

In cases where the geranium essential oil is used inside, it is diluted with honey, jam, and always washed down with plenty of tea with lemon. The recommended rate is: 1 drop 2 times a day after meals.

Essential oil of geranium in cosmetology: geranium oil for the skin, face and hair

Geranium oil is effectively used in perfumery and cosmetics, primarily due to the fact that it is non-toxic and non-irritating to human skin. In the production of cosmetics it means to be an complement for bath and shower soaps, lotions and creams, and is often used as a base when men's perfume and cologne a created.

At home, essential oil of geranium can enrich the usual cosmetics (2 drops per 30 ml of base). It is suitable for all skin types, but particularly beneficial effect has on *oily skin and skin with age-related changes.* Due to the fact that, firstly, has a clear anti-inflammatory and antiseptic effects, and, secondly, promotes rapid renewal of epidermal cells. Moreover, geranium oil normalizes the sebaceous glands and thus prevent the emergence of new inflammation, making the skin smooth and youthful. It can also be applied in pure form to the affected area. Adding it in hair care products, essential oil of geranium helps to get rid of dandruff and is effective for everyday use.

Essential oil of geranium: contraindications

Geranium oil can not be used in children under 6 years of age, pregnant women in the first two trimesters of gestation, as well as people of all ages on an empty stomach. Furthermore, the application rate should not exceed three weeks.

St. John's Wort Oil: Composition and healing properties. St. John's wort oil in cosmetics. Indications and contraindications for the use of essential oil from St. John's wort.

In the woods, on the meadows and fields around, you can see a whole bucket of beautiful green shrub with yellow stars like flowers and beautiful leaves. This is St. John's wort that has long been known as an assistant in the fight against many diseases. This plant is found in the Mediterranean, in the middle lane and close to the northern latitudes.

For a long time St. John's wort was the first medicine in Europe. Our ancestors said like that: 'without flour does not bake bread'' and ''do not cure the disease without St. John's wort''. Many people were drinking it instead tea, thereby preventing many diseases. And if you have any ailment - the first thing is to drink a decoction from this solar grass. This herb can be used for all diseases, so to speak, from head to toe. It treats nerves, and stomach, liver and kidneys, and skin damage. And healers claim that St. John's wort imbues man with solar energy, it helps improve mood and relieve depression and boredom.

Ancient people believed that St. John's wort drives away evil spirits and helps to safeguard the house from them.

The composition and useful properties of St. John's wort

Wort contains: triterpene saponins, flavonoids, tannin, essential oils, vitamins C and E, anthraquinones, minerals and other biologically active substances.

Infusions and decoctions from St. John's wort is used as an antiseptic and astringent for intestinal catarrh, rinsing for inflammation of the mucous membranes of the mouth and throat, to lubricate the mouth in stomatitis.

Preparation St. John's Wort oil: the first recipe

Wort is used as a therapeutic agent in many types of disease. One of them – wort oil, which is prepared in several ways. Moreover, oil of St. John's wort can be prepared with your own hands. To do this, take 20g. of fresh flowers and pour 200 ml of olive oil, over. Ingredients must infuse for 40 days. The oil is then filtered through filter paper ,coffee filter or gauze. According to the experience - through cheesecloth is fastest way.

The use of St. John's wort oil

Indications for use of St. John's wort oil: *peptic ulcer, stomatitis, periodontitis, pharyngitis, as well as diseases of the bile duct and kidney stone disease.* Have a great analgesic and anti-parasitic actions.

Preparation of St. John's Wort oil: second recipe

The second recipe is that you must take half a cup of fresh chopped leaves and flowers of St. John's wort and pour on them almond oil. You can take as sunflower, olive or linseed oil. Insist for three weeks, wring it well and drain. Keep the oil in a cool place.

The use of St. John's wort oil

This oil is very good for *burns of varying severity, tightening long-healing wounds, ulcers and abscesses.* With it you can also treat ulcers, inflammation, boils, breaks on the mucous membrane of the mouth, on the lips from the common cold.

Caution: St. John's wort oil if is properly prepared has a distinct reddish-brown color. Experts advise to get a quality end product, to use it freshly.

St. John's wort oil in cosmetics

St. John's wort oil is excellent for oily and combined skin, subjected to dehydration. It prevents loss of moisture, is able to normalize the composition of the hydro-lipid layer of the skin. Also, this oil is used as the antimicrobial agent, it has an active anti-inflammatory, soothing. St. John's wort oil has been successfully used for the care of the porous skin and skin with problem fat areas. It cleans, whitens and reduces pores. Effectively for abrasions and white acne.

Also, St. John's wort oil has a regenerative effect, helps the formation of a beautiful tan, it relieves neurodermatitis and allergies. If you have problems with dandruff - St. John's wort oil is rubbed into the scalp. In this case it will also contribute to a more rapid hair growth.

The therapeutic effect of St. John's wort oil

In St. John's wort oil there are many volatile products, so it is so effective in treatment. In conjunction with flavonoids, resinous substances and other valuable components of oil it has beneficial effect on the skin.

For internal use: it relieves cramps, regulates the filtration ability of the kidneys and peripheral circulation. With St. John's Wort oil you can also soothe stomach pain. It has a diuretic effect, and disinfecting substances contained in the oil help to prevent cystitis. When bites of cats and dogs wounds do not heal for a long time, it can also help.

To enhance the effect of St. John's wort oil is better to add to it cypress oil (10 ml. to 10 drops of cypress oil).

When St. John's wort oil is better not to apply:

a) If you are in the sun for too long.
b) If you are working in institutions related to radioactive radiation.
c) If your work is connected with high temperatures.
d) In pregnancy.
e) At elevated body temperature.
f) Hypertension.

To avoid problems, wort oil is best to be used internal in combination with other oils, which means the amount should be at least 80% of other oils.

Contraindications

St. John's Wort – is an slightly toxic plant, so too big dose ingestion can cause discomfort in the liver, and the bitterness in the mouth. It can cause narrowing of the blood vessels, so persons with high blood pressure should be careful with drugs from St. John's wort. St. John's wort is also "not friendly" with some medications, so it should not be taken simultaneously with contraception, AIDS drugs, after organ transplantation, during rehabilitation.

Wort is considered a natural antibiotic, so it is not combined with artificial antibiotics, as well as with antidepressants. Simultaneous administration of these agents can lead to dizziness and migraines.

Another contraindication for receiving St. John's wort are- pregnancy and lactation, as well as sensitivity to sunlight. **In any case, a doctor's advice never hurts.**

Avocado oil: structure and advantageous properties. Uses of avocado oil. Avocado oil in hair cosmetics, eyelashes, face and hands.

Avocado oil - the result of the mechanical pressing of fruit pulp of avocado, also known as the "alligator pear". This is one of the most environmentally friendly vegetable oils, which by its nutritional value, chemical composition and taste characteristics is superior to most other useful products. Homeland of avocado, evergreen tropical plant, is considered Chile, but today it is grown commercially in the United States, Central America, some South African countries, Australia and New Zealand. For the production of avocado oil manufacturers select only the best, and most importantly only ripe fruits, and then the pulp is separated from the skin, bone and gently squeezed under strict temperature control. Then, using a centrifuge oil is separated from the fruit pulp and the liquid is pumped into stainless steel tanks. Thus prepared avocado oil, should have an emerald green.

Avocado oil: structure and advantageous properties

Avocado oil - it is no exaggeration to storehouse of nutrients, vitamins and trace elements. In it contain balanced amount of protein, carbohydrates, saturated and unsaturated fatty acids. Furthermore, it contains such components as lecithin, amino acids and phosphatides.

With regard to vitamins, for example, vitamin F in avocado oil is several times more than in the fish oil. Vitamin F is a set of polyunsaturated fatty acids, which are directly involved in the development of human cells and normalize blood circulation. This vitamin is also necessary to adjust the fat metabolism and removes toxins, radionuclides and heavy metals.

No less important to the health and preservation of youth is vitamin E content in avocado oil, and it exceeds olive oil by more than 5 times. It slows down the aging process of cells and is necessary as a warning factor for atherosclerosis, arthritis, cancer and prevents thrombus formations. Vitamins from group B, in avocado oil, are represented by vitamins B1, B2 and B3. They are able to have a beneficial effect on the human nervous system, as well as improve blood composition.

In addition to vitamins avocado oil contains a wide list of relevant micro- and macro-elements (iron, iodine, potassium, calcium, cobalt, magnesium, manganese, copper, sodium, phosphorus, zinc, silver, etc.) that must flow into the human body for its normal functioning.

The use of avocado oil

Regular avocado oil eating elevates mood, improves efficiency, charging with vital energy and helps to cope with psycho-emotional disorders, such as insomnia, headaches. Moreover, it enhances the potency in men, eliminating the frigidity of women and, in some cases, can cure some forms of infertility.

Uniqueness of avocado oil consists in that it does not have contraindications and may be easily incorporated into the diet of pregnant women, lactating women and children.

Avocado oil in cosmetics for hair, eyelashes, face and hands

Avocado oil, through the optimal combination in it of vitamins B, D, E, F has a positive effect on dry and peeling skin, nails, weak hair. Moreover, it is effective to both forms of use: internal and external.

For internal use with avocado oil are advised to fill salads, use it for sauces, meat and fish dishes, pastas and a variety of dishes from see foods. For external administration, use avocado oil added to various cosmetic products. In addition, you can enrich your favorite cream, balm, lotion or shampoo alone. Example: to 10 grams of the foundations in the form of a cream (tonic) or per 100 grams of shampoo (conditioner, hair balm) add 10 drops of avocado oil.

Due contained in it of polyunsaturated fatty acids in high concentrations, avocado oil restores the protective function of the epidermis and increases the local immunity of the skin. And, due to it constituent of fat-soluble vitamins A and E, avocado oil confer antioxidant and regenerative properties.

Acting on the hair, avocado oil removes their fragility, it helps solve the problem of split ends and gives hair a natural shine. It is useful for colored and weakened hair by chemical exposure.

The pure avocado oil may be used by combining it with other types of vegetable oils, it is used as a basis for combination with other oils.

Recipes for avocado oil in cosmetics

a) Face mask with avocado oil for aging skin:

Ingredients: 1 tablespoon of avocado oil, essential oil of sandalwood, chamomile, orange and rose- 2 drops of each. The solution is impregnated in paper towels and applied on problem areas of the skin for up to 30 minutes in the morning and evening. **Indications:** skin loose with age-related changes, the damaged or inflamed skin, fine wrinkles around the eyes. The result is noticeable after 5 treatments.

b) Avocado oil for massage:

Used for massage avocado oil is able to provide anti-cellulite effect and soften hardened skin areas. To enhance the effect in 2 tablespoons of the basis in the form of avocado oil is recommended to add 2 drops of essential oil (lemon, juniper, fennel, cypress or rosemary).

c) Avocado oil for nails:

To strengthen the nails and cuticles, avocado oil is connected with any vegetable oil (almond, apricot) in the ratio of 1 to 1, or add to it (at the rate of one tablespoon), 2-3 drops of essential oil of lavender, patchouli, chamomile or lemon. The mixture is applied to the nails daily and massage the nail and cuticles until the oil is completely absorbed. The procedure is recommended prior to application of decorative lacquer.

!!!Avocado oil is even used as an oil for tanning. He has excellent safety features and it protects the skin from harmful UV rays.

Linseed oil: healing and medicinal properties, treatment. Linseed oil in cosmetics, for the face, body and hair.

Flax - is one of the first crops, which people began to grow in agriculture, and it happened in ancient times - in Egypt, India and other countries.

The healing properties of flaxseed oil

The healing properties of flaxseed oil are known in our country for a long time. As a food product, this oil has been indispensable: it can be use for cooking meatless dishes, and during the holidays, as it is very tasty and fancy cakes with the addition of linseed oil takes on a special flavor and aroma.

Medicinal properties of linseed oil

Medicinal properties of linseed oil and seed are also known for a long time, and folk medicine has always used them to treat *ulcers, cuts and wounds, pain reduction, relief of heartburn, expelling of worms.*

In our time, when the linseed oil finally is able to really expose its medicinal properties it became known more, and today its well helps us fight disease, to restore and maintain health.

Of course, only throw results of modern research, we could learn that eating linseed oil reduces the risk of serious diseases such as stroke - more than one third, and unsaturated fatty acids useful in it are more than two time higher than in the fish oil. Therefore, flaxseed oil protects us from *diabetes, hypertension, coronary artery disease, atherosclerosis, and many other chronic diseases.* It is known from our ancestors, that in the old days when it was flaxseed oil on each table, the percentage of these diseases was many times lower, and ordinary people were hardly aware of such diseases. And vegetarians who do not eat even fish, can also easily compensate deficiency of unsaturated fatty acids using linseed oil.

The useful linseed oil

Today, nutritionists often recommend eating flaxseed oil for people with disorders of fat metabolism, as it is very easy to digest, and promotes the breakdown of saturated fat. This property of flaxseed oil is very important for those who want to *lose weight.*

There are a variety of diseases, when the body is in dire need of polyunsaturated fatty acids, omega-3 and omega-6 - and linseed oil have a lot of them. For women, these substances are particularly important in the diet of pregnancy - this will ensure the correct formation of the brain of the child. Linseed oil also supports normal female hormones, it facilitates postmenstrual syndrome and improves the well-being during menopause.

With what is useful to use linseed oil

Especially useful to combine flaxseed oil along with fresh vegetables, potatoes, so it is recommended to fill a variety of salads and vinaigrettes. Any porridge, first or second dish will become more valuable and nutritious by adding flaxseed oil to them.

Fresh cheese is tastier and healthier, if you add in place of sour cream and sugar to it, the oil and chopped parsley. So the body can get the daily rate of unsaturated fatty acids, it is enough to eat only a few spoons of flaxseed oil per day, adding it to the various dishes - you can even add it to your yogurt and kefir.

Flax seeds contain about 50% oil, and it is obtained by cold pressing - so it retains all its medicinal and nutritional properties. Color of linseed oil can be different: golden, yellow, almost brown - it depends on the degree of purification, and its calorie content is very high - about 900 kcal per 100 g of linseed oil. Contains some minerals, and the main of them is phosphorus, but useful vitamins are a lot - it's vitamins A, E, F, K and group B.

The fatty acids in linseed oil

Essential components of linseed oil are fatty acids represented by alpha-linolenic - 60%, linoleic - 20%, oleic - about 10%. Another 10% falls on the share of other fatty acids. All these acids are necessary for us to live, but they are not synthesized by the body - *we can get them only with food.*

You must know that Omega-6 is found in other vegetable oils: olive, sunflower, soybean, mustard, but Omega-3 - only in flaxseed. The deficit of omega-3 fatty acids leads to deterioration of brain function, reduces the concentration of attention and speed of thought processes.

Treatment with linseed oil: folk recipes

Flax seed oil helps to reduce swelling; It is recommended in various neurological disorders and diseases: *stress, insomnia, depression.*

The work of the entire digestive system will come back to normal, if you regularly use linseed oil: *it will improve the work of the liver, gastritis and colitis will dissapear, depart heartburn and constipation.*

For the treatment of *constipation* is recommended: a mixture of linseed oil (1 tablespoon) with a small amount of natural yogurt or honey. Drink this mixture in a refrigerated form, an hour before bedtime.

Constant use of flaxseed oil as food provides us with a strong immune system and protect against some *cancers - including colon and breast cancer.*

Doctors recommend patients who underwent surgery or weakened after a long illness, taking flaxseed oil to help the body recover. In such cases, the reception of course can last 2 or 3 months in this form: *1-2 tbsp. per day - this dose is divided into several stages.*

For children and adolescents linseed oil is recommended for growth and development, especially in the period of *intensive training.*

Children and adults with chronic diseases of the *respiratory system* should be constantly adding flaxseed oil to the diet - *1-1.5 tablespoons/daily,* since it promotes the development of substances that protect the bronchial mucosa of inflammation. For children with *weak immune* is recommended this therapeutic mixture: *flaxseed oil (3 tsp) mixed with sugar (1 tsp.) – take 1 tsp. 2-3 times per day.*

In diseases of *the kidneys and gallbladder, thyroid, nervous disorders and sexual dysfunction* is also advised to regularly include in the diet the flaxseed oil. Most of nutritionists believe that to achieve success in *weight loss* is possible only with the help of linseed oil, if it is partially replaced with animal fats, but do it consistently: *20 ml of flaxseed oil per day will help to get rid of superfluous kg.,* oil reduce appetite, because it will stimulate the saturation center, and comply with any low-calorie diet will be much easier. Besides, linseed oil accelerates the movement of food in the gastrointestinal tract so that fewer calories are absorbed in the intestine - this also promotes *weight loss.*

It should be noted that flax oil is not subjected to heat treatment (if you do not add it to baked goods), to enable it to keep all the vitamins, and not to lose useful and healing properties. It is also possible to use linseed oil with honey - so its positive effects will increase.

Linseed oil in cosmetics for face and body

Of course, this amazing healing oil could not miss estheticians: it is often recommended for *skin care* - both normal and problematic, as well as to improve the *condition of hair and nails*.

Due to its *antioxidant, anti-inflammatory, regenerative and wound-healing properties, flaxseed oil moisturizes, nourishes, softens and protects the skin of the face, hands and body.* That is why it is recommended for *daily skin care* - it maintains its tone, rejuvenates, protects against sun, wind and frost, is used to treat warts and corns.

Linseed oil for hands

For rough and flaky skin of the hands there are very good mixture of linseed oil with honey, lemon juice and egg yolk. You must just 15-20 minutes to massage the skin with linseed oil in this mixture - such a procedure is also well softens and eliminates peeling.

Linseed oil for face and body skin

A few drops of linseed oil added to a night cream, will enhance its features and make it more effective.

Excellent mask for dry skin with the addition of linseed oil can be prepared from the pulp of fresh cucumber and sour cream. To 1 tablespoon of the mixture you must add 1 tablespoon of linseed oil, and put a mask on your face for 15 minutes. After using this mask complexion becomes fresh and inflammation and redness disappear.

For oily skin are suitable mask with cottage cheese and sour cream (1 tablespoon), egg yolk and linseed oil (2 tsp). The mask must be applied on clean and moistened skin, and hold for 15 minutes.

Normal skin also feels much better after applying the mask with linseed oil. For it, is necessary to mix: *one ripe tomato or a strawberry, add egg yolk and flour (1 tsp.) linseed oil (2 tsp.), and mix it until a homogeneous mass is obtained.* The mask is applied to the face for 20 minutes.

Flaxseed oil can be used to care for any skin type, as well as for *aging, fading, peeling skin*; it is often used for general massage - in pure form or in admixture with other oils.

Linseed oil for hair

For hair care flaxseed oil is also perfectly: for this purpose it can be used both externally and inside. If you use *1-2 tablespoons of flaxseed oil a day,* your hair will always be in good condition.

To improve the hair, linseed oil, can be applied to them as well as on the scalp, massaging it in a circular motion with light movements. This is very useful for dry and colored hair, as well as for fatty ones, as the oil leads to normal activity of sebaceous glands.

Strengthens hair such mask: linseed oil (50 ml.) and glycerin (30 ml.), apply direct to the hair overnight.

When buying flax oil, choose one that is grown without the use of chemical fertilizers - it is called organic. Flaxseed oil should be sold only in containers of dark, preferably black, otherwise it will be useless - under the influence of light and heat, it is oxidized, and can even cause poisoning.

Mustard oil: structure, benefits, features, treatment, and contraindications. The use of mustard oil in cosmetics for the face and hair.

Mustard oil - the result of the cold pressing of the seeds of Sarepta (blue-gray), white or black mustard. Cold pressing method involves a temperature that not exceeding 50°C. This eliminates the likelihood of the raw material decomposition and preserves most nutrients: enzymes, vitamins and amino acids. Different mustard seeds contain 35 to 47% of essential oils and have a different flavor, color and aroma.

The oil produced from the seeds of black mustard, have light yellow color with a saturated characteristic odor and taste. References to it are found even in the most ancient European cultures. It was used for cooking, for the treatment and even for soap making.

Oil from the seeds of white mustard is yellow and have a spicy taste. It was popular in India and China, primarily due to its medicinal properties. In these countries, white mustard was called "warming" and "destroying leprosy"

Mustard oil: composition, properties and use

The essential mustard oil by 40% consists from alilmustard oil, that provides burning taste and specific aroma of the famous mustard dining. His carrier is a glycoside: sinigrin, substance which under the influence of hot water is split into alilgorchichnoe butter, sugar and sulfur and magnesium salts. In addition, mustard seeds contain glycerol and various fatty acid (erucic, ominovaya, linoleic, linolenic). Thus, for example, linoleic acid belongs to the group of omega-6 in combination with linoleic acid could have a salutary effects on humans bodies. The complex of these two acids *normalizes fat metabolism, hormones, strengthens the immune system and improves the function of the digestive organs.* Their regular replenishment have an positive effect on the *cardiovascular system, preventing the development of atherosclerosis and reducing cholesterol levels.*

A large number of biologically active substances are part of the mustard oil, which on a daily basis should act in the human body. These are *vitamins A, D, E, K and B group; volatile phytosterols, glycosides, chlorophyll.*

Vitamins in mustard oil

1. Vitamin A (retinol) is an antioxidant and provides a full development of the organism. It improves the condition of the organs of vision, promotes regeneration of cells of the epidermis, and supports the immune system.
2. Vitamin D maintains the level of calcium and phosphorus in the blood microelements, improves thyroid, prevents the development of a number of skin diseases. Its ample presence in the human body is considered to be a preventive measure for multiple sclerosis and the occurrence of malignant tumors.
3. Vitamin E - a fat-soluble vitamin that has anti-inflammatory and healing properties. Its amount in the mustard oil (as well as the amount of vitamin D) is much greater than commonly used in our country oil sunflower. Vitamin E normalizes blood clotting and prevents the formation of blood clots, strengthens the walls of blood vessels, and also affects the activity of the reproductive system. Vitamin K is known as "antihemorrhagic vitamin" for its ability to prevent bleeding associated with low blood clotting. In addition, it plays an important role in calcium absorption and bone tissue, it is useful for the smooth operation of kidneys. Vitamins form group B presented in mustard oil mainly vitamins are: B6, B3 (PP) and B4. The first is considered a "female" vitamin, as it supports normal hormone balance and the state of the female reproductive system, second is required for proper operation of the digestive organs, and the third - "choline", is part of the lecithin and improves brain activity. In addition, the B vitamins are involved in various metabolic processes: energy, fat, carbohydrate, protein and water-salt.

These biologically active substances such as phytosterols ("plant hormones"), volatile chlorophylls and sinegrin have clearly marked *antibacterial and anti-tumor properties.* They will help the cardiovascular, endocrine and digestive systems and more phytosterols will also improve the condition of the skin.

Mustard oil: indications and treatment with mustard oil

Mustard oil - a drug with a broad spectrum of prophylactic and therapeutic effect. The indications for its use are:

1. Cholelithiasis, cholecystitis, hepatitis, cirrhosis of the liver;
2. Hypertension, atherosclerosis, anemia;
3. Pregnancy and lactation;
4. Prostatitis, BPH, prostate cancer;
5. Diabetes;
6. Different degrees of obesity;
7. Nervous system diseases;
8. Eye diseases;
9. ENT diseases.

For external use, mustard oil is advised for the treatment of *arthritis, rheumatism, sciatica.* It is well relieves tension in the muscles and ligaments after considerable physical exertion. In folk medicine *it is used for faster healing of cuts and injuries.*

Contraindications for mustard oil

Despite the many beneficial properties of mustard oil, it has a number of contraindications. Firstly, because of its component of erucic acids, adversely affecting the myocardium, *people with diseases of the myocardium mustard oil can include in the diet only after consultation with a cardiologist.* Secondly, it is necessary to limit the use of mustard oil to those who have observed *hyperacidity or gastric ulcer and duodenal ulcer.* Third, contraindication is an individual intolerance of components from mustard oil and highly sensitive skin in cases of extern use.

Mustard oil: uses in cosmetics for the face and hair

In cosmetology mustard oil is effective in getting rid of *acne, seborrhea, herpes, psoriasis and other skin lesions.* It is easily and quickly absorbed into the skin, it nourishes, softens and moisturizes. Thanks to contained in it vitamins A and E, it protect the skin cells against premature aging, especially associated with excessive exposure to ultraviolet radiation.

When mustard oil rubbed into the scalp. It prevents hair loss, and even their premature graying.

Mustard oil can be combined with other essential oils, using it as a base, and can be added to shampoo to wash your hair (just prior to application).

Lotion for body care. Ingredients: 1 tablespoon of mustard oil, other cosmetic oil (almond, peach) 1 tablespoon, sandalwood, lavender and ylang-ylang 1 drop. Suitable for daily care of the face and body after taking water treatments.

Hazelnut oil: composition, properties. Hazelnut oil in cosmetics and cooking: recipes.

Hazelnut oil gain popularity only in the 70-ies of XX century, but its flavor and medicinal qualities were quickly appreciated by the consumers long before 1970.

Useful proteins in the oil are as much as in the meat , but the digestibility of the protein is much easier. Vitamins and minerals in it are too much - more than many long-known and used vegetable oils.

Saturated fat in hazelnut oil are very few, so it is almost completely absorbed by the body, in 100%; if you regularly use it for food, then the *chances of getting heart disease and blood vessels are reduced by more than half.*

Dieticians and beauticians called hazelnut oil *source of beauty, health and good mood.*

Of course, it's an oil and has a very pleasant taste: sweet and soft, with a delicate aroma of hazelnut.

The composition of the hazelnut oil

If we talk more about the composition of hazelnut oil the amount of such unsaturated fatty acids not found in any other vegetable oil: they are in it 94% - mainly oleic acid and linoleic.

Among vitamins - E, C and group B; there are almost all essential amino acids; mineral composition - sodium, zinc, cobalt, iron, magnesium, phosphorus, and calcium.

As already noted, hazelnut oil is well absorbed by our body, and vitamin E content is so high that it has a very beneficial effect on the *thymus*, the normal operation of which depends the state of our immune system.

Energy value of hazelnut oil

For strict vegetarians who do not consume meat, hazelnut oil is a complete source of protein and carbohydrates; it can be safely used even for those who are prone to the *accumulation of excess weight and diabetes.* Energy value, both from the nut and the oil, produced from it, is quite high, and therefore it should be used in *heavy physical exertion, loss of strength, and exhaustion as a restorative remedy for increasing endurance and improving adaptive abilities of body.* In hazelnut extract have been founded substances having *anticancer properties.*

The properties of hazelnut oil

Hazelnut oil has anti-inflammatory and regenerating effect, and hence wound healing properties that can be used in the treatment of various diseases and in cosmetology.

Astringent and toning properties of this oil are also used in folk and official medicine. It can help you improve the bowels, liver and rid the body of toxins and even parasites - such as some kinds of worms.

Due to the high content of polyunsaturated fatty acids, hazelnut oil is used successfully in the treatment and prevention of many cardiovascular diseases and prevents atherosclerosis. Sodium, potassium and calcium, which are part of the hazelnut oil, *maintain normal blood pressure* and help to *strengthen the bone.*

Hazelnut oil is also useful to maintain *visual acuity and reduces seizure activity of the brain in epilepsy;*

Hazelnut oil in cosmetology

Manufacturers and cosmetics specialists (dermatologists, beauticians) also like to use hazelnut oil, either in pure form or as a base oil in cosmetic compositions and mixtures with natural aromatic oils.

Finished cosmetic benefit only when it is added to the hazelnut oil: it is introduced into the mask, creams, shampoos, conditioners, etc.

Especially effective is the oil of hazelnuts in the care of problematic oily and combination skin: *it cleans and tightens pores, removes acne, cures boils and abscesses.*

It is used for skin care around the eyes, and the treatment of rosacea - spider veins and "asterisks" on skin. All effects of aggressive environmental influences are eliminated with hazelnut oil: caused by the sun, wind or frost, redness, irritation, scaling - in these cases it acts very effectively without causing any side effects.

As an anti-aging tonic the component of hazelnut oil is used in the home creams and masks: it smoothes existing wrinkles and prevents the appearance of new ones.

With regular use of hazelnut oil as a massage for the skin of the whole body you will get healthy appearance, decrease the appearance of cellulite; hair become stronger and no longer drop if regularly to make masks for hair with hazelnut oil on the scalp.

Traditional recipes with hazelnut oil

1. The easiest way to use oil - put it on the fingertips (you can add other oils, both basic and essential oils in a certain proportion) and with light massaging movements rub into the skin of the body.

2. For foot massage oil should be mixed: hazelnuts (4 parts), sesame (2 parts), St. John's wort and calendula (1 part). Take 1.5-2 tablespoons prepared mixture and add thereto lavender oil and tea tree (5 drops). Apply the mixture on the feet and massage until is completely absorbed.

3. To improve the complexion, you can use the following application: to 1 tsp. of hazelnut oil add a couple of drops of oil of cypress, orange or spruce. The mixture is applied to the tips of the fingers and with light massaging movements rub into the face skin. The acne can be overcome by using a different combination of oils: to the oil of hazelnuts (1 tablespoon), add eucalyptus oil (5 drops), sage (3 drops) and cypress (2 drops). Daily apply a mixture of these oils on the pre-cleansed face.

4. Eliminate rosacea problem will help application with hazelnut oil (1 tsp.) and lemon essential oil, cypress and lime (3-5 drops). This mixture should be applied on wet cloth and apply to the places with the vascular pattern. The result is only achieved at a sufficiently prolonged use.

5. Those how have normal skin can make a mask for the face with hazelnut oil (1 tablespoon), walnut (1 tsp.), strong black tea (1 tsp.), milled wheat and grain (1.5 tsp.). All the ingredients are mixed thoroughly and applied on face for 20-30 minutes. Wash with warm water. Make mask 2-3 times a week, until the skin becomes more fresh and supple. After that, you can do it once a week - to maintain the achieved results.

6. Just to clear the skin, is enough to moisten the swab in warm water, then wring out and put on it a few drops of hazelnut oil - pure or mixed with other oils, and gently rub the face.

7. To strengthen the hair, oil should be applied to their roots in following mixture: hazelnut oil with egg yolk 1: 1. Do this before washing hair, hold for 15 minutes and then wash your hair with a mild shampoo.

Hazelnut oil can not be called cheap, but the price is offset by taste and usefulness. To preserve its taste as long as possible, it is better to store it in the fridge - otherwise it can become rancid.

Oil hazelnut in cooking

The cooking oil is used in *sauces, dressings, baked goods, in dishes from meat and fish* - it gives them the original nutty flavor, but it should be added gradually, otherwise the taste will be too bright.

The fish should be only lightly sprinkled with hazelnut butter before serving; if you add oil to the mashed potatoes or pasta, their new taste will surprise you, and the home and guests will appreciate it.

You can mix the hazelnut oil with other oils - peanut or walnut - it softens its rich taste. For frying, this oil is not suitable. It is best to add this oil to salads.

Cinnamon oil: composition, properties and use. Use and treatment with cinnamon oil. The essential oil of cinnamon in cosmetology and cooking.

On from the exotic island of Sri Lanka (Ceylon) is native evergreen shrub Cinnamomum Ceylon, better known to us as Cinnamon. From it, is produced not only a popular pastry spices but and the aromatic oil. The percentage of oil content in the bark, leaves, stems and young shoots is less than 1%, so for the production of essential oil on a commercial scale a large amount of raw materials required. Plantation of cinnamon trees exist in India, Vietnam, Egypt, Brazil, as well as on the islands of Java, Sumatra and Madagascar. However the most high-quality oil is produced in the historic homeland of cinnamon - Sri Lanka from the finest soft bark, pale yellow or brown. Removed from the dried bark of young branches and shoots, crushed, soaked in the sea water and the resulting infusion is then subjected to steam distillation.

Cinnamon Essential Oil: composition

Initially, cinnamon oil has a yellow-golden color, characteristic odor of cinnamon and hot aromatic taste. Later, cinnamon oil undergoes a process of oxidation, and therefore becomes resinous and darkens. The composition of cinnamon essential oil varies in addiction from what part it is produced, from the bark or leaves of plants. For the first main component (80%) is cinnamic aldehyde, whereas the second contain a similar amount of eugenol per unit. For this reason, cinnamon oil from bark from eponymous bush is advantageously used in cooking, and then to create a cosmetic or perfume as an auxiliary component for making them. Created from the cinnamon leaf essential oil of cinnamon goes only to the manufacture of fragrances for cosmetics, detergents, soap and tobacco.

Features and benefits of essential oil of cinnamon

For most people, cinnamon oil is associated with something warm. It seems no coincidence, because cinnamon is able to warm up, both physically and emotionally. The aroma of cinnamon essential oil eliminates the fear of loneliness, feelings of isolation. At the same time it relaxes, calms and even inspiring. With the help of cinnamon oil you can create an atmosphere of mutual trust, eliminate feelings of envy for others and compassion for yourself. On physical layer the cinnamon essential oil improves metabolism, stimulates circulation, normalizes the gastrointestinal tract, reducing flatulence and eliminating constipation. It is recommended for colds and flu.

The essential oil of cinnamon is effectively as part of warming massage mixtures, capable of neutralizing the poison from insect bites and helps with pulmonary forms of food poisoning, as it removes intoxication syndrome. Cinnamon oil is also used in dizziness and nausea. It accelerates the healing of injuries and the disappearance of bruises and abrasions. In the presence of inflammation in the mouth and bleeding gums reduces inflammation and eliminates odor. It is believed that the essential oil of cinnamon enhances sexual desire, due to the fact that stimulates blood circulation in the pelvic organs in men and women. Furthermore, women may use this oil to reduce menstrual pain.

Cinnamon oil is good for the sport, it increases the efficiency, helping to heat up faster and easier to endure physical stress.

The use and treatment with essential oil of cinnamon

Treatment with cinnamon oil varying in ways how it is applied: externally, internally, by inhalation, comprising a massage and even through incenses. Cinnamon essential oil blends well with other types of essential oils, in particular: spruce, mint and orange in proportions of 1 to 1.Concentrated cinnamon oil is used only for application to the field of insect bites, in other cases it is usually combined with something, for example with vegetable oil (15 ml of base to 3 drops of cinnamon), for rubbing against rheumatism, for getting rid of skin parasites, and for the treatment of bruises and abrasions.

-A mixture of the base oil (one tablespoon), 1 drop of cinnamon, orange and eucalyptus oil can help relieve muscle pain, has a warming effect and stimulates circulation.

-If you have bleeding gums, add in a glass of boiled water 2 drops of oil and rinse your mouth several times a day.

With essential oil of cinnamon you may do hot inhalation. To do this, take a container with hot water and add 5 drops of oil, tilted your head on it, covered with a large towel and deeply inhale vapors for 3-7 minutes. At the same time during the procedure, the eye must always be closed. Hot inhalation are especially effective for colds, general malaise and loss of strength.

For internal use: cinnamon oil (1-2 drops) is added to a teaspoon of honey, jam or marmalade. It is recommended to drink herbal tea after use of oil. As an alternative to remove the first signs of a cold, it is possible to prepare a therapeutic compound based on dry red wine. To do this, heat up 1\2 glass of wine, dissolve it in 1 tablespoon of honey, 3 drops of essential oil of cinnamon, cloves and cypress. All mix thoroughly and drink.

The essential oil of cinnamon in cosmetology

Essential cinnamon oil is widely used in cosmetics, especially in view of the fact that it is replete with antioxidants and tannins, able to reduce inflammation. Beauticians use it to cleanse the skin.

In addition, cinnamon stimulates the metabolism and improves blood circulation, as an excellent prevention and treatment of the initial stage of cellulite. It is also believed that the essential oil of cinnamon eliminates paleness of skin, improves the complexion and gives it a healthy look. At home, the oil of cinnamon can be connected to your favorite cosmetic product at the rate of 2 drops of oil to 15 ml of base. Thus, you will enrich your makeup, adding to it, even more useful features.

In addition, if you are prone to hair loss, you can add essential oil of cinnamon in the shampoo and conditioner, thereby providing additional power hair.

The essential oil of cinnamon in cooking

The oil of cinnamon is used in cooking much less frequently than ground cinnamon or cinnamon rolls (the dried inner bark of the cinnamon bush). However, it can be used in the preparation of various dishes. As a rule, cinnamon is a good addition to sweet dishes (cakes, drinks, deserts), alcoholic cocktails, wine, coffee. Sometimes it is combined with poultry, beef or fish. In all its manifestations cinnamon raise appetite, improves digestion and has a healthy effect on the gastrointestinal tract.

Sandalwood essential oil: structure, benefits, use and treatment with sandalwood oil. Sandalwood oil in cosmetics, for the face, hands, nails and hair

Essential oil of sandalwood - a product with a rich history that goes back more than 4000 years ago. References to it are found even in ancient texts written in Sanskrit. In India, it was used during religious rituals, in the smoking candles to relax and go into a meditative state. In Egypt, sandalwood oil was used for embalming. In addition, the healers of ancient civilizations know about the healing properties of this oil. To date, the essential oil of sandalwood, still remains the main oil for meditation as well as an indispensable ingredient in the perfume and cosmetics industry.

Essential oil of sandalwood: composition

Sandalwood essential oil - the result of long-term water-steam distillation (from 48 to 72 hours), of the pre-soaked chips of sandalwood that have at least 30 years. Chips are obtained both from its timber and from the root system. Homeland of sandalwood is considered tropical regions of South Asia, and best of all, this plant feels at an altitude of 600 to 2,500 meters above sea level. Due to the fact that, to obtain 100 kg of sandalwood essential oil requires about 1 ton of bark-wood, and due to the fact that the resources of this type of tree severely depleted, sandalwood oil cost is quite significant.

Up to 90% from sandalwood oil is santalol component, in addition to it there are: teresantalol, santal, santalon, santa and santenon. According to its consistency is thick, viscous, with a yellowish tinge and grass-wax aroma.

Sandalwood oil: the use, application and treatment. Properties of sandalwood oil

The use of sandalwood essential oil is quite diverse. It is used to treat people for flavoring alcoholic beverages, perfume and cosmetics industry, as well as a repellent (eliminates burning, pain and insect bites).

Let's start with the fact that sandalwood oil has pronounced antiseptic, antibacterial and anti-inflammatory properties. It is equally help with external skin infections, diseases of the respiratory and digestive systems.

Essential oil of sandalwood has antitussive and expectorant effect, so it is effective in bronchitis (including chronic), sore throat, rhinitis, SARS and other diseases, accompanied by a dry cough. Useful for the genitourinary system, as it helps to cope with cystitis, urethritis and vaginitis, and has a diuretic effect. When it is used regularly, it normalizes the menstrual cycle, enhances the potency in men and an increase sexual desire in women, it is considered a kind of erotic stimulant.

Sandalwood oil is not just considered a major oil for meditation. Thanks to its special properties, it relaxes and soothes, brings calm in stressful situations, eliminates tearfulness, while improving strength and body toning. It is believed that the oil of sandalwood opens creativity, talent, gives a sense of personal completeness. It also helps to cure headaches and handle insomnia. Sandalwood oil may be used for inhalations (3 drops to a small tank with hot water) and aroma lamps (7 drops to 20 square meters), added to the bath (9 drops per 200 liters water) and for massage (8 drops per 30 gram base), making lotions and compresses. With it you can even enrich wine bouquet, based on the proportion of 5 drops of oil to 750 ml of wine. Like the perfume added to an alcoholic drink, it will give a slight flavor of "east" direction.

Sandalwood oil is contraindicated in pregnant women and people with chronic kidney disease.

Sandalwood oil in cosmetics for the face, hands, hair and nails

Essential oil of sandalwood for centuries was used to maintain both female and male beauty of different ages.

Young girls and boys used sandalwood oil to get rid of acne, it is well regenerates and soothes the skin cells, it is recommended to owners of oily skin type.

In later years, this oil is effective for rejuvenation, eliminating sagging. It refreshes and gives the skin tone and tightens facial contours.

In cosmetic properties of essential oil of sandalwood also includes its ability to whiten the skin, give it a natural color. In addition, it is an excellent moisturizer. When mixed with any natural vegetable oil obtained lotion is used for irritated skin after shaving.

Thanks to its special delicate action, sandalwood oil is suitable even for sensitive skin around the eyes, as well as other areas with low-fat skin.

Sandalwood oil - the perfect remedy for hair care. The use of sandalwood oil helps to stop loss, eliminate dandruff, strengthen and stimulate hair growth. It can be added to shampoos, conditioners and balms, and can be applied to the tips of the comb and just comb your hair in such a way. Such a complex effect will restore the health of your hair and give them shine.

Sandalwood oil is effective for the prevention and fight against varicose veins. It improves circulation and blood circulation, tones the muscles of the venous wall, thereby preventing the occurrence of such unpleasant disease.

For cosmetic purposes essential oil of sandalwood can enrich the most commonly used means - creams, face masks and body lotions and so on (at the rate of 4 drops to a 20 gram base), and can be used in pure form, combining with other types of essential oils.

For example, for an anti-aging procedure, make a mask with following composition: 1 drop of sandalwood, vetiver 3 drops, 3 drops of incense, jojoba oil-1 tsp.. The resulting composition is applied to skin, left for 15 minutes, after which the excess oil is removed using natural rose water.

In the presence of acne, sandalwood oil is better to put in a dot on inflammation place several times a day.

Essential oil of pine: the benefits, indications, the use and treatment with pine oil. Pine oil in cosmetics for the face, hands and hair.

Essential oil of pine - the result of the water-steam distillation of various parts (needles) The evergreen trees, pine, are native to northern strip of the country. This light, fluid and volatile liquid is colorless or have slightly yellowish color. Its structure includes components such as pinene, sylvester, cadinene, karen, bornylacetate, terpineol, and resin acids. To obtain one kilogram of pine essential oil is required not less than 500 kg of fresh needles. In retail 10 ml of 100% pine oil is, depending on the manufacturer, about 3 dollars.

Essential oil of pine: the use, treatment and indications

The healing properties of pine oil are known for a long time. Even in ancient times it was used for *bleeding, open wounds, burns of varying severity and frostbites.* They treat rheumatism, scurvy. With it, you can get rid of the lice and deduce fleas in domestic animals. It was also believed that the essential oil of pine is able to get rid of the *pessimism and overcome nervous exhaustion.*

According to modern research, the basic properties of pine oil is analgesic one, helps to overcome cough and has antiseptic effect. As adjuvant treatment is recommended for:

- asthma;
- SARS, flu, rhinitis, sinusitis;
- diseases of the upper respiratory tract;
- diseases of the urinary system;
- eczema.

The special composition of essential oil of pine *normalizes pulmonary ventilation, and minimizes respiratory failure*, is an excellent antitussive, especially when coughing in smokers. It also regulates *blood pressure, relieves headaches, dizziness; removes and eliminates the tremor.* Precise dosage of pine oil can act as a diuretic and anti-edema means. It is noticed that regular use of pine oil reduces *erectile dysfunction in men and increases the potency.* Experts advise to use pine oil during *rehabilitation after a lengthy illness and serious injury.*

If necessary psycho-emotional correction, essential oil of pine *energizes, gives strength, focuses and improves response.* At the same time it makes people *less aggressive and irritable, gets rid of suspiciousness.*

Contraindications for pine oil

Pine oil is contraindicated in **hepatitis, glomerulonephritis, as well as during pregnancy.**

Essential oil of pine: application

Pine essential oil, it is used both internally and externally.

For internal use, pine oil is added to tea or make a drink based on water and honey with 5 drops of oil, ½ teaspoon of honey, a glass of warm boiled water.

For extern use, essential oil of pine have a little more indications. These include *compresses, rubbing, massage, inhalations, baths and oil burner.*

To make a compress on the joints, burns, wounds and other injuries: use a piece of ordinary cotton fabric, which is soaked in the solution *(per 100 grams of water add 5 drops of oil),* slightly wring out and apply to the sore spot. The timing of the procedure in case of imposition of a hot compress is: two hours, and in the case of cold compress - 20 minutes. In grindings oil-base is combined with essential oil of pine and rubbed into the skin on the affected areas. Trituration massage is analogue, and helps with *inflammation in the muscles, connective tissues in nerve.* It improves *blood circulation, affects the respiratory and lymphatic systems.*

The most rapid penetration for essential oil of pine inside the body provides massage. In this situation, oil is also connected to the base fluid and applied to the skin during massage. Such tandem has a positive effect on the *central nervous system, respiratory system, blood circulation, and also heals the liver and the intestine.*

For the inhalation, pine oil is added to a bowl of hot water, then lean over it, covering your head with a big towel, and take a deep breath. Inhalation procedure lasts on average about 10 minutes, with the mandatory 30-second intervals. When you do inhalation of steam, eyes should be kept closed. It can be used as a *cleansing steam bath for the face.*

For taking a bath with pine oil (add 5 drops per bath) is also recommended to add sea salt, honey, cream or the classic bubbles. You can combine water treatment with a light self-massage. *Recommended bath time: less than 20 minutes.*

Oil burner is used primarily for flavoring premises. For this purpose, a mixture of essential oil and water in the reservoir are heated by a special evaporator candles. Essential oil of pine is able to rid the room from *cigarette smoke, the smell of animals.* It also decontaminates *the air and is a sort of antiseptic.* Moreover, the oil burner with pine oil favorably affects the mental and emotional state. Dosage: for the treatment of 5 square meters, you will need 100 grams of water and 2 drops of pine oil.

Oil in cosmetics for the face, hands and hair

For cosmetic purposes pine oil is used as an enriching component of the various means: *creams, emulsions, tonics, masks:* 3 drops per 5 ml base. It is believed that the essential oil of pine has an *anti-aging effect, regenerates the skin and increases the protective function of the epidermis.* Effective in *acne, seborrhea, pigmented spots, for the prevention and treatment of scars.*

Essential oil of pine has beneficial on hair, it can also be added to shampoos, conditioners and balms. It strengthens the hair, removes dandruff and helps to combat alopecia (hair loss).

On the basis of pine oil you can make cosmetic ice to wipe the face, neck and décolleté. For this: *mix a teaspoon of honey or cosmetic cream with 200 ml of water and 2 drops of oil, frozen in portions and subsequently use in the morning and evening.*

Shea butter: properties and composition. The use of shea butter in cosmetics and at home: creams and masks.

The earth is very rich and offers us everything that is necessary for a full and happy life. If only more, we have learned to accept these gifts, and intelligently manage them - but that is another question. Using the gifts of nature, we can secure a wise and good nutrition, as well as long stay young, healthy and beautiful.

Shea oil, is precisely such a wonderful gift of nature. Is a seed oil of unique African tree - in other continents such trees do not grow.

The Latin name of the tree is- Butyrospermum parkii or karite tree. Lives shea tree for a long time - nearly 300 years, and the healing properties of its fruits have long been used by African nations. This tree is very strong - it has a thick bark, and it is always alive and green - on the spot of falling leaves immediately grow new.

The composition of shea butter

Shea butter is dense, has a light cream color, and consists mostly of triglycerides - substances produced by fatty acids - oleic, stearic, palmitic, and unsaponifiable fats. Unsaponifiable substances found mainly in plants and does not react with alkalis, as fatty acids. In the small quantities, shea oil also contains linoleic, linolenic, myristic acid, carbohydrates and proteins.

That union of fatty acids and unsaponifiable fats makes shea butter (shi) so popular in cosmetology. More 70 years ago, scientists noticed that the African nations that use Shea butter for the skin, almost do not know what is a skin disease, and their skin for a long time remains remarkably elastic and smooth.

Properties and treatment with shea butter

In cosmetology, shea butter has been used for more than 20 years, and cosmetic products, in which it is affiliated, are the most competitive in today's market.

Shea butter has a strong regenerating properties and protects the skin from the sun, so in Africa from children to adults, all use it.

Only way to get oil is cold-pressing procedure: it gives a very dense, non-homogeneous, white or slightly creamy, with a slight nutty flavor oil. It becomes liquid at body temperature - even at 35 ° C, so it is easy to use fo a massage - it spreads in the skin and is quickly absorbed.

Anti-inflammatory properties of shea butter allow its use for the treatment of skin problems - *pimples, sores, dermatitis, and rub into the painful joints and muscles, remove the swelling.*

Although this oil does not have a vasoconstrictor action, it can be used to successfully treat a runny nose - and here, too, work anti-inflammatory properties.

Shea butter by Estheticians is called -transport, thanks to its ability to penetrate deeply into the skin and deliver in layers, various useful ingredients of cosmetic products. These components can be easily connected with the oil, and, getting into the skin, just as easily and quickly released from it. It is widely used in the *care of lips, facial skin, hair and is a part of sun protection cosmetics and cosmetics for tanning.*

Through regenerating properties of unsaponifiable fats, oil stimulates *the synthesis of collagen, and is recommended for mature and aging skin.* The protective properties of the oil due to triglycerides: *the barrier function of the skin when applied is amplified.*

The use of shea butter in cosmetics

If you use shea butter regularly as a standalone tool, it *improves the complexion, skin texture becomes denser, the tone increases, decreases the depth of wrinkles and the skin becomes elastic.* Therefore, shea butter is often a part of the anti-aging cosmetics.

Pregnant women are recommended to use it for the prevention of stretch marks on the skin.

The protective properties of the oil are also expressed in its *moisturizing effect.* One hour after application it reached the maximum moisturizing and protective effect that persists for 8 hours, protecting the skin from the effects of a plurality of aggressive external factors. In addition, shea butter effectively eliminates *dryness and irritation of the skin, nourishes it with vitamins and prevents early aging.*

Shea oil at home

Shea oil can be used in different ways in the home. It can be applied *on the entire face, like a mask, and even in the area around the eyes,* after 30-35 minutes just wash with a little warm water.

Melt the oil directly in the hands, or drive across the face a small quantity - it will melt and be absorbed into the skin. Lubricate the skin with shea oil in summer and in winter, when you are in the sun, or on the street in the cold and windy weather, and do not just face and neck - apply shea butter on all *exposed areas of the body.*

You can mix shea oil with other oils - for this purpose it is necessary first to melt it in a water bath. With it you can also easily prepare *homemade creams and masks.*

Creams based on shea butter

- Cream for dry, aging and sensitive skin: 2 tsp. of shea oil melt in a water bath, then add the almond oil (4 tsp.), remove from the heat and stir until completely cool. While stirring, add essential oils - camomile blue oil (3 drops) and lavender oil (2 drops). The cooled cream put in a glass container and refrigerate.
- Recipe cream with shea oil: similarly preparing the cream with the other ingredients. Shea oil, as well as in the first case, 2 teaspoons, and when it is melted, add avocado oil and jojoba oil (1 tsp.), and macadamia oil (2 tsp.). After removing the mixture from the heat, and stirring, add rosemary oil (2 drops) and rosewood oil (3 drops). Let cream to cool down during the mixing; then put in the fridge.
- Prepare a regenerating night cream is a little more complicated and require more ingredients: First you have to mix in a separate container- 1 tsp. of rose water without alcohol and 1 teaspoon of aloe vera gel. In another capacity it is necessary to melt the beeswax (1 tsp.), putting it in a water bath, then add shea oil (2 tsp.), olive oil (1.5 tablespoons). Instead of olive oil you can take the peach, apricot or almond oil. Stir the mixture until the ingredients are unite completely, and then add one capsule of vitamin E from pharmacy - open the capsule and pour into a mixture - and lecithin (on the tip of teaspoon) and mix further. Without ceasing to interfere, add mix with aloe vera gel, rose water, remove from the heat and stir until then, until the cream has cooled completely - you can take a small mixer. Again, in the process of mixing, add the essential oils - chamomile (3 drops) and tangerine (2 drops). Ready cream store in the refrigerator in a glass jar.

Masks based on shea butter
All mask with shea oil soften and nourish the skin.

- You must take one dried lemon peel and grind it in a coffee grinder to get flour for the preparation of nutritious and energizing facial masks. To the crude egg yolk you must add 1 tsp. from this flour, stir, close the container and leave for 20 minutes. You can then add melted shea oil and walnut oil - 1 tsp.. Mix everything again and apply on face for 20 minutes. Rinse with warm water.

- Mask with shea oil and avocado suitable for drier skin: Crush the avocado flesh, take 2 tablespoons from it, and add to it 1 tsp. of melted shea oil, jojoba oil and the same amount of liquid honey. Mix carefully, apply on face for 15-20 minutes, then rinse with warm water. If you do not have an avocado, you can take a banana or persimmons, and if the mixture turns out too thick, add a little egg yolk.

Shea oil for Hair

Shea oil can be added to any home nourishing and softening facials products, as well as for hair. Apply melted butter especially on the roots, and wrap with a hot towel for half an hour - during which time the hair will absorb everything that is good for them. Then wash your hair as usual.

You can also apply shea oil after washing your hair, when they dry up: a small amount of oil will give hair shine and revitalize them.

Shea butter does not cause any unpleasant reactions, and its surplus will simply not be absorbed.

Contraindications for shea butter

However, not so long ago, scientists found that this oil also has contraindications - though quite rare: the sensitivity to latex. The fact is that in the composition of shea natural has been founded latex.

Cosmetics with shea oil often is not cheap, but is it possible to save your youth and beauty!

Essential oil of fennel: the use, application, properties and treatment. Fennel oil in hair cosmetics, facial skin, body and hands.

Essential oil of fennel - a result of the steam distillation of fennel seeds of the plant whose homeland is considered the ancient Persia and India. Its fruits contain from 2 to 6% of essential oils and to produce 1 kg of such substances is required not less than 20 kg of seed. The composition of the essential oil includes components such as anethole, fenhol, camphene, pinene, limonene and phellandrene. At the same time it has a sweet and slightly spicy flavor, vaguely reminiscent of anise.

Fennel oil: the use and application

Fennel essential oil has properties that are able to exert a healing effect on a wide variety of components of the human body. It can help you to carry out a *comprehensive cleansing, remove toxins*. It has a *slight diuretic and laxative effect and stimulates the digestive system, eliminates constipation, reduces bloating.* Such oil is particularly useful for those who are interested in eating excessively and drink a lot of alcohol. *Fennel - a proven folk remedy for a hangover, it tones and normalizes the liver, kidneys and spleen.*

Fennel oil is useful for women of different ages, **as mimics the hormone estrogen and thus activates the endocrine glands and the production of its own estrogen.** This facilitates the *premenstrual condition, relieves pain during menstruation, and helps in solving problems associated with menopause.*

During lactation fennel oil helps to *increase lactation*, therefore, is a part of most homeopathic remedies that stimulate the production of milk. In addition, it is believed that the essential oil of fennel *improves sexual desire*, both in women and men.

Properties of fennel oil

Fennel has a pronounced *antifungal* activity. It is proved that with regular sanitation of the facilities (*at the rate of 2 drops per 5 square meters*), the content of fungi in the environment is reduced by 5 times.

It is also known the positive effects of essential oil of fennel on the human nervous system. Its flavor gives *strength and courage, helps get rid of obsessive fears and complexes, gives a sense of inner stability and independence, and also gives a serene feeling of freedom.* On assurances of some centenarians - fennel is able to *prolong life.*

The use of essential oil of fennel is quite diverse. In addition to use with food or beverages, it is used topically for *massaging, for enrichment of cosmetic preparations (masks, lotions, tonics, gels, etc.), for application of compresses, bath preparations, applications to gums, as well as inhaled (oil burner).*

Fennel Oil for Treatment

Essential oil of fennel can be used as an additional health-improving agent for various diseases. It has *expectorant and anti-inflammatory effect*, and therefore it is recommended for the prevention and treatment of *SARS, influenza, pharyngitis, bronchitis and pneumonia.*

By acting on the cardiovascular system, fennel oil *lowers blood pressure, removes arrhythmia, improves cardiac conduction.* Fennel also has the ability to *dissolve kidney stones and stimulate the activity of the digestive system*, it is advised to use the essential oil in patients suffering from gastric diseases.

As improvised means in the home medicine cabinet, fennel oil helps with *nausea, vomiting, colic and the usual hiccups.*

Contraindications to the use of fennel oil

Essential oil of fennel is not recommended for pregnant women, children under 5 years of age and people suffering from epilepsy.

Fennel oil in cosmetics for hair, face, body and hands

Fennel oil is a strong antioxidant, and all its derivatives are invariably endowed with the same properties. It slows down the *aging process and has a powerful anti-aging effect on the skin, smoothing fine lines and improving the elasticity of the upper layers of the epidermis.* It helps to cope with the problem of *cellulite, tones the skin*, makes it more elastic stomach, hips and bust.

Essential oil of fennel is able to solve teenage problems, eliminating *acne* and preventing the emergence of *new pimples.*

Fennel oil can be added to any cosmetic means for hair (shampoo, conditioner, hair mask), facial skin, body or arms skin. Can be used in combination with other oils to create recipes home cosmetics.

1. Lifting mask for the face and décolleté.
   Ingredients: 1 egg yolk, 1 tablespoon of white clay, jojoba oil- 1 tablespoon, fennel essential oil 1 tablespoon, rose essential oil- 1 tablespoon, 1 tablespoon of neroli essential oil. Thoroughly mix the clay, egg yolk, base oil, after add essential oils. Facial mask is applied on clean and dry skin, before application relax in the horizontal position (in order to prevent skin sagging under the weight of clay) – time of application 30 minutes. Then rinse with water of contrasting temperatures, first with warm, then with cool. Recommended course - 1 month, once every three days. The base can be replaced with jojoba oil, if desired, any other vegetable: almond, grape seed, olive..
2. Anti-cellulite massage oil.
   Composition: 50 ml of base oil, essential oil in proportion of 5 drops each - fennel, patchouli, lime, grapefruit. All ingredients are mixed immediately before use. Ideal for problem areas of the body. In connection with any kind of clay is suitable for carrying out the procedures for aging skin.
3. Mask for face and hands

Ingredients: quince 1 piece, egg yolk 1 piece, cottage cheese 1 teaspoon. essential oil of fennel 3 drops. Grind throw a blender the quince, add cottage cheese, egg yolk and oil. The mixture should be like paste. Apply it on the face or the back of your hands, wash off with warm water after 15 minutes.

4. Anti-Aging Eye Cream on the basis of fennel oil.
   Ingredients: any baby cream- 1 tablespoon, fennel essential oil- 4 drops, myrrh essential oil 4 drops, you must heat for a few seconds the cream, add the oil and liberally apply the mix on the eyelids before going to bed.

5. Cream for rough skin of hands and elbows.
   Composition: any baby cream 1 tablespoon, mint oil 3 drops, geranium oil 2 drops, essential oils in proportion of 1 drop each (fennel, grapefruit, incense). Mix well, apply as needed. The cream can be stored in a glass container in the refrigerator.

Essential oil of fir: composition and properties. The use and treatment with fir oil.

Essential oil of fir, or just fir oil is obtained by water-steam distillation of needles, young branches and cones from fir or white fir. Fir is an evergreen tree from the pine family, which reaches 30 meters high. Like any other tree of this family, fir can exist only in pure air and in the absence of any industrial pollution and, therefore, the essential fir oil - is an environmentally friendly product.

Essential oil of fir: composition and properties

Fir oil - a colorless or yellowish-greenish liquid, light and with fluid texture with a fresh-resinous pine aroma. This oil is used as a raw material for synthesizing medical camphor. It contains tannins, carotene, ascorbic acid and tocopherols. Due to its high biological activity, fir oil has an valuable *cosmetic, curative, disinfectant and anti-inflammatory properties,* which mankind has been using for more than one century. Its special properties are also associated with *bactericidal and antiviral effect.* Fir can suppress *staphylococcus, respiratory infection, and rod-shaped bacteria*, which is why in the coniferous forests of the air is particularly pure and fresh. And, as a rule, after the visit in the forest there is a feeling of lightness and vigor.

Fir oil contributes to the successful treatment of *bronchopulmonary pathologies*, in particular the purification of the trachea and bronchi, reduce total *intoxication* and reduce *inflammation*. It is also effective as a prophylactic agent for susceptibility to acute respiratory infections and influenza.

For people who underwent serious and prolonged illness, the last sessions of radiation, for those who need fast acclimatization to the new environment as well as for those who need to recover from the emotional stress, fir essential oil may be just what they need. It is recommended for heavy physical activities and to maintain the normal functioning of the cardiovascular system. It have an interesting effect on a person's blood pressure, *aligning reduced by lowering the high and absolutely without altering the normal.* In addition, we should know that a part of the elements of pine oil regulate glucose levels in the serum. It have property to *activate the gonads*, both female and male, and have a positive influence on the activity of the hormone system.

The use and treatment wtih pine oil

Fir essential oil can be used both: pure form (internally and externally), and by inhalation, as a main constituent of aromatherapy, but also as a main component for the preparation of ointments and salves.

At the use of pine oil inside, its peculiarity consists in the fact that it is not subjected to a process of decomposition in the gastrointestinal tract and into the blood, and is directed into the painful lesions of the body.

For external use, pine oil primarily *disinfect wounds, abrasions, scratches, it prevents small wounds fester.* The composition of essential oils of fir includes 35 different elements that help to restore the skin's structure and nourish its with useful micronutrients. Suitable for treatment of most skin disorders, including *acne.*

When connecting pine oil with melted pork or goose fat, a fat raccoon or badger, it turns out the healing ointment, which is used in the treatment of already heavily suppurating wounds, eczema and trophic skin ulcers.

It treat *sciatica, low back pain, arthritis.* Penetrating into the joint tissues, oil improves *blood circulation and lymph flow, thus removing pain and restoring normal nutrition of cartilage tissue.*

Fir oil against toothache

Fir oil will help in case of emergency to remove *toothache.* To do this, soak a swab of cotton wool or bandage in the oil and apply to the aching tooth for 10 minutes, repeat the process after some time. It is also effective for the treatment of *periodontal* disease, but this rate is extended up to 20 applications and if you want you may repeat it after a couple of months.

Baths with essential oils of fir

Inhalation and aromatherapy with pine oil are relevant during epidemics of *catarrhal diseases*, in the treatment of *sore throat, bronchitis*. It can clean the space inside house, it is believed that its actions are similar to scents such as frankincense, lavender and eucalyptus. For fans of aromatherapy: it can be directly added in the bath, just a few drops of oil in your water. Such a bath calms the *nervous system, relieve fatigue, add forces and strengthen the immune system*. Moreover, the regular "fir" bath will improve *skin tone, get rid of wrinkles and sagging*. They are useful for the prevention of *gynecological and urological diseases*. If the time spent in the bath increased to an hour, you will give an opportunity to relax your *tense muscles and can easily fall asleep*. In this case your sleep will *be quiet and deep*.

Contraindications for fir essential oil

Essential oil of fir, with any method of use is not recommended for pregnant women and people with intolerance to fir. Note also that with the treatment of pine oil is categorically not compatible alcohol . Otherwise, the treatment effect will not be achieved.

Like most other essential oils, fir oil is decomposed by exposure to sunlight and is oxidized by atmospheric oxygen. Therefore, to preserve all curative properties keep it tightly sealed and in a dark place.

Essential oil of bergamot: properties, use and contraindications. Essential oil of bergamot in cosmetology.

There in the family of Rutaceae and genus Citrus, one very rare specimen called "bergamot". This plant can be found only in one of the Italian coast, where it grows in its original form. However, the creator of bergamot – man, scratches bitter orange and orange in resulting obtained a great evergreen plant with a great aroma. Italians are very proud of these trees growing near Bergamo, because only the soil and climate of the place make it possible to grow the fruit with the most vivid and rich aroma.

Bergamot essential oil is obtained from the fruit, leaves and flowers of this plant. Yield is very small, so the oil is valued very highly.

The properties of essential oil of bergamot

Bergamot oil has so many useful properties. It is used as an *antispasmodic, sedative, anti-inflammatory agent,* as a means to massage the skin, as well as an *antiseptic.*

Like all essential means, the bergamot oil helps to recover energy: *it can enhance communication skills, strengthen imagination and creative thinking.* It can be called an aphrodisiac because bergamot essential oil is used as a means of *enhancing libido for partner.*

It has useful properties which helps *normalize the secretion of the sebaceous and sweat glands,* the ability to narrow the pores of the skin.

In folk medicine, bergamot oil is used as an *antifungal and parasiticide agent, anti-inflammatory* for diseases of the upper respiratory tract, as well as to reduce the temperature.

The use of essential oil of bergamot

1. Aromatic lamp: 3-7 drops per session.
2. Aromatic medallion: 1-2 drops.
3. Forbath: 4-8 drops of oil mix with a spoon of milk or cream, add in bath of warm water (45 degrees), to take no more than 15 minutes.
4. Steam room :5 drops per use for flavoring steam.
5. Rinse for throat: in 100 ml of warm water , dissolve 2 drops of bergamot oil and 2 drops of tea tree oil. This facility also helps in the inflammation of the oral cavity.

Essential oil of bergamot in cosmetology

1. For massage: 5-7 drops of bergamot oil mix with 10g of the base oil, used for body massage.
2. The additive for cosmetics, add 1 to 5 drops of bergamot oil in any cream, tonic, mouthwash or a face mask. It will enrich any means, giving them new qualities.
3. Cleanser for skin: Dissolve 1 tsp. of grape oil and 5 drops bergamot oil and the same oil of thyme. This tool should be rubbed into the skin on a daily basis at any time of the day.
4. Body oil: take the sweet almond oil (50ml), add 5 drops of bergamot oil, 5 drops of lemon oil, 3 drops of neroli oil and 1 drop of rosemary oil. This tool has a refreshing and cooling effect.

5. Means for oily skin: In 75 ml of distilled water, add 15 ml of glycerol, stir 5 drops of geranium oil and 5 drops of bergamot oil and 3 drops of sandalwood oil. Mix well, apply on the face at night. The tool removes the shine, it normalizes fat metabolism of the sebaceous glands.
6. Means for hair care: Apply to massage brush one drop of oil of bergamot and just comb your hair in different directions. The hair will become shiny and unforgettable aroma.
7. The means for the hands and nails: Apply 1-2 drops of bergamot oil on your hands, spread over the entire surface, including nails. Your hands will get an excellent tool for power and cooling.

Bergamot oil for the body

Bergamot oil – is a good assistant for strengthening *the brain*. It will acquire a clear focus and clarity of thought, will help you to *structure the information received during the day*. For example, before an exam or interview is recommended to drop in aroma locket oils of grapefruit, bergamot and lavender. Even at work, you can *fight fatigue*, using the aroma lamp, or simply dropping oil of bergamot on a piece of foam soaked in water and placed on a table. At lunchtime, you can massage the neck and shoulders with massage oil with the addition of bergamot - *courage will return*.

Treatment with oil of bergamot

The classic recipe: in a tablespoon of honey, drip 2-5 drops of bergamot, use 30 minutes before eating. It will help get rid of inflammation in *"ENT" area, bladder, reproductive organs*. This agent is used to *reduce the temperature, to enhance appetite and destruction of intestinal parasites*. According to rumors, **this tool helps to break the habit of smoking.**

The essential oil of ginger: the use, structure, properties and applications. Ginger oil in skin and hair cosmetics.

Ginger, meaning in Sanskrit "horned root", it is a herbaceous plant of the ginger family. It has long stems that can reach one and a half meters high, and the orange-yellow flowers. Homeland of Ginger is considered to be India, but this plant grows with success in Japan, China, Ceylon and other countries in Southeast Asia and Central

America. The ideal conditions for its growth - a warm, humid climate and a height of not more than 1,500 above sea level. However, it is grow, as the garden, and as a houseplant - in flower pots or special boxes.

The only valuable part of ginger is it root. It has many useful properties and *may be consumed.* There are two kinds of roots - *black and white.* The difference between them is reduced to the method of processing. White (Bengali) Ginger is thoroughly cleaned with a brush, scalded with boiling water, rinsed in 2% sulfurous acid or bleach solution and then dried in the sun. Black (Barbados) ginger is not cleared, but simply washed and dried. Due to the fact that black ginger undergoes less processing it has taste and aroma of a tart, spicy and full-bodied.

The use of ginger oil

Ginger root can be used in different ways. It is actively used in medicine, pharmacy, cosmetics and cooking. Since the content of essential oil are not large, in rhizome from 1 to 3%, to obtain 1 kg of natural oil requires at least 50 kg of dried rhizome. The essential oil of ginger in the middle can be purchased at the price of 10 dollars for 10 ml, but the cost can vary significantly depending on the country of origin. It is believed that the prime ginger oil is produced on the Malabar Coast from India.

The use and composition of essential oil of ginger

The essential oil of ginger contains large amounts of minerals and vitamins. These micro-and macroelements, magnesium, phosphorus, calcium, sodium, iron, zinc, potassium, combined with vitamins C, A, group B, and in the complex have a significant revitalizing effect on the human body.

The properties of essential oil of ginger

The main properties of essential oil of ginger include its ability to provide an *anti-inflammatory and antiseptic effect.* It is successfully used for the treatment of diseases *of the nervous system and diseases of the musculoskeletal system, such as arthritis, arthrosis, different degrees of stretching.* Essential oil *improves memory, helps to get rid of fear, apathy, reduces aggression and causes a person to believe in themselves and their own strength.* It also helps with *headaches, migraines and nausea caused by nerve disorders.*

In addition, since ancient times ginger root is considered an aphrodisiac, able not only to maintain a long time libido, but also to cure female frigidity. In the 19th century in European countries existed even so-called "candy harem", which is based on ginger.

The use of ginger in any form should be restricted to pregnant women, nursing mothers and people with diseases of the gastrointestinal tract.

The essential oil of ginger in cosmetology

1. Gingerbread for the skin and hair oil

The essential oil of ginger - an indispensable tool in the composition of many face masks, creams, tonics for the skin. Interacting with the skin, it has a *stimulating effect, improves blood circulation, has anti-aging effect, removes some of its defects*. When applied to problem skin, ginger oil stops the inflammatory processes of different nature, occurrence from bacterial and viral rashes to premenstrual and herpes. It increases the tone of the upper layers of the epidermis, reduces pores and normalize fluid balance of skin. When ginger contact with head skin it *nourishing hair roots, strengthens them and helps to cope with the problem of hair loss and baldness.*

Ginger hair mask, you can easily prepare yourself. For this it is necessary to rub ginger fine and then connect with any vegetable oil (sunflower, olive, castor oil). The resulting mixture is applied to the scalp for 15-20 minutes and then wash your hair with your usual shampoo.

Ginger is used effectively in *anti-cellulite programs,* as it perfectly warms and moisturizes as well as for the treatment of scars and prevent stretch marks (striae).

Ginger essential oil is added to the bath, in the massage oil, for compresses and is used for inhalation. In addition, it can be added to your favorite beauty products for the face, body, hair, including shampoos and shower gels, at the rate of one drop per tools serving.

How to prepare ginger oil at home

At home, you can cook ginger oil for culinary delights and extern applications.

To prepare ginger oil for salads, meat dishes or a basis for a variety of sauces, cut ginger into slices and warm up in the required amount of vegetable oil. Preference is better to give to olive, peanut or corn oil. Ginger is fried until it acquires a dark color. To prepare the "inedible" ginger oil, cut ginger, filled with oil (in this case, your choice will depend on your individual requirements) and put in a dark place for 21 days. For containers it is recommended to use a glass bowl as it does not emit harmful substances that can change the properties of the oil. The resulting ginger oil can be used *for warming and anti-cellulite massage, for grinding the back, for the treatment of painful joints, to reduce the swelling of feet.*

Walnut oil: structure, properties, application, and treatment. Walnut oil in cosmetics for skin and hair, tanning and slimming.

Walnut since ancient times is considered to be the fruit of wisdom and intellectual development. Even in ancient Persia among scientists has been a statement recorded in a medical treatise, the fruit of a walnut - is the brain, and the oil pressed from it - the mind. Unfortunately, recent studies have not found this reasonable evidence, but nevertheless the useful walnut and its derivatives, no one will undertake to deny.

Walnut oil is obtained from its core by cold pressing. It has a beautiful amber color, original taste and rich nutty flavor. By virtue of such a pronounced smell of walnut oil it should not be used to create a subtle aromatic compositions.

Walnut oil: structure and properties

Walnut oil is a storehouse of nutrients and trace elements. It comprises: polyunsaturated fatty acids, particularly linoleic and linolenic; carotenoids and retinol, vitamin A; Vitamins E, C; B vitamins, as well as micro and macro elements, such as iodine, iron, calcium, magnesium, zinc, copper and others. This oil record the content of vitamin E and omega-3 and omega-6, which make up 77% of the substance.

The use of walnut oil

Thanks to its unique composition, walnut oil can be used in cooking, in cosmetics and medical purposes. Its regular use has on the body *rejuvenating effect, increases vitality, removes radionuclides from the body, reduces the level of cholesterol in the blood, strengthens the protective functions of the body and increases its resistance to radiation.*

Treatment with walnut oil

Walnut oil is recommended as an adjuvant treatment for the following diseases:

1. mucosal inflammation;
2. oncological diseases;
3. tuberculosis;
4. chronic arthritis;
5. chronic colitis;
6. otitis;
7. diabetes;
8. constipation;

9. ulcerous stomach and bowel disease.

As a prophylactic agent, it is indispensable for people who have a predisposition to *atherosclerosis, cardiovascular disease, liver disease,* as well as for those who have violated the metabolism. My advise is to use during the recovery period after the transferred operations and severe diseases.

Among other things, it is also a kind of aphrodisiac. Part of the special oil enzyme *increases blood circulation in the area of the genitals and stimulates the production of sperm in men.*

It is useful for pregnant women, as included in its composition vitamin E, that plays an important role for the proper development of the fetus and reduces pregnacy manifestations.

Walnut oil for topical application *promotes rapid healing of wounds, cuts, burns and inflammations.* It is also effective against *varicose veins.*

The use of walnut oil in cooking is not very popular in our country, but to have such a habit is such a hard thing. It will complement and improve the *flavor of salads* with fresh vegetables, can become a highlight of the *cold sauce.* On it, you can fry the meat and add as baking at home cooking.

Walnut oil in cosmetics for skin and hair

Walnut oil is widely used in cosmetics, thanks to vitamins and minerals, suitable for all skin types, moisturizing, toning and nourishing the skin. It is a component of a large number of creams, balms and means for hygiene of body. Used in its pure form, it is easily and evenly distributed in the skin, it is absorbed quickly and leaves skin soft and silky. Especially recommended to owners of *sensitive and prone to irritation of the skin,* as has the property to *calm and cool.* Ideal for *dry skin, eliminates cracks in the body and lips.*

Walnut oil, at the expense of any contained polyunsaturated fatty acids and antioxidants (vitamins A, E, C), has a *regenerating and rejuvenating properties,* respectively, can be used as a means to combat **skin aging, in particular to prevent and get rid of fine wrinkles.** With regular application to the body, it tightens the skin, leaving it smooth and supple.

Walnut oil is used for *strengthening hair.* For this purpose, it is possible not only to include in your diet, but also to do on it the basis of "home" mask. For example, with the addition of eggs and honey. *Composition mask:* walnut oil 2 tablespoons, 1 egg piece, honey 1 tsp.. All the ingredients are mixed. The resulting mixture rub into the scalp, wrap in a warm towel and leave for half an hour. After, wash your hair with your usual shampoo. The mask will have a *stimulating effect on blood circulation, hair will get extra food to become strong, healthy and supple in the installation.*

Walnut oil for tanning

If you do not trust the cosmetic for suntan, pay attention to the natural walnut oil. It can be taken with food, thus protecting the body and skin from the *inside*, and can be applied *directly* to the body as a normal suntan oil. In addition, it is believed that this oil is effective for the *preservation and maintenance of already acquired tan.* It can *improve the color and extend the "life" of your bronze skin.*

Walnut oil for weight loss

Walnut oil is appreciated by those who are struggling with *excess weight,* because it is a great fat burner and diet product. It is an excellent *source of energy, vitamins and other nutrients,* and it is very easily absorbed by the body. It is an indispensable product of many healthy diets.

It can be added to food, and can be consumed on an empty stomach (30 minutes before meals) ,one teaspoon (adult) up to 3 times a day. **Course application is unlimited, there are no contraindications.**

Essential oil of cypress: properties, use, indications and contraindications. Cypress oil in cosmetics for skin, hair, hands and nails.

Cypress, aka Cupressaceae - evergreen coniferous handsome, reaching a height of about 30 meters. In the wild form is found in the Mediterranean, and for ornamental and medicinal purposes is grown in many countries with warm climates. The ancient Greeks and Romans considered very durable the cypress tree, and used it for the construction of ships and other household needs, as well as cased their home, temples and caves. In addition, almost all parts of the plant are used for medicinal purposes.

Properties of cypress oil

Cypress oil is obtained from its fruits - nuts and leaves and small branches. It contains odorous liquid with terpene, pinene, camphene and terpineol, and some acids. These components determine the remarkable properties of cypress essential oil. It is able to kill many pathogens, restore emotional state, have beneficial effect on skin and hair when applied topically.

Benefits and indications for cypress oil

Everyone knows very well that cypress oil relieves *nervous tension*, the bath with the oil remove *the sense of fatigue and relieve insomnia*. When irritability and other emotional disturbances appear in the human sphere, it will help to calm down and gain emotional balance. You can also use cypress oil as an *aphrodisiac* - to enhance the sensitivity of *erogenous zones* and to stimulate blood circulation in the pelvic organs. In this sense, it is effective even for people who are not of very young age.

In folk medicine cypress oil is used for *varicose veins, hemorrhoids, menopause problems, infectious and broncho-pulmonary diseases.*

In the tradition of oriental medicine, in particular in Tibet, remained till our time the use of cypress oil as a *cleaning agent*. It is used to treat *diarrhea and to reduce sweating*. Bioenergists called cypress oil "protector". It is able to prevent the outflow of power from human and protect chakra from all contamination: the evil eye and spoilage. It recommended it the night to put the vessel with water and 3-4 drops of aromatic oil or lamp near the bed for a more restful sleep. During the day you can wear aroma medallion or apply oil on the temples and wrists several times a day.

This is especially useful for people who have a lot of work to communicate with other people, or a large amount of time they spend in the public.

Cypress oil for the skin

Cypress oil is able to solve many problems of the skin. It will help in *pustules, remove warts and papillomas, cleanse skin of old dead cells.*

If the skin is prone to irritation and if it came in the form of a capillary pattern "stars" - you can use this oil both internally and externally, of course, after talking to your doctor.

Massage with cypress oil helps *get rid of cellulite and make the skin more elastic.*

As a rule, in all cosmetic products for the sweating of the feet can also be found cypress oil, since it is a well neutralizer of the unpleasant smell of sweat.

Cypress oil for hair

Cypress oil when applied to the scalp *strengthens the hair follicle, stops hair loss, normalizes the sebaceous glands, and when applied to the hair itself helps them to get rid of the fragility and acquire live shine.*

Contraindications for cypress oil

If you are using oil of cypress you must be careful : if you are pregnant women, children under 12 years of age, people with cancer, with symptoms of mastitis, increased blood clotting, thrombophlebitis, post infarction states, as well as allergic reactions to it components.

Recipes with cypress oil

Before giving practical recommendations, I note that anyone can do on their own any funds for the skin and hair using a variety of essential oils. However, it should be remembered that the cypress oil is particularly successfully combined with *cedar, pine, lavender and tangerine oil.*

1. Aromatic medallion: 3-6 drops.
2. Aromatic lamp: 2 drops per 5 square meters.
3. Anti-cellulite bath: 2 drops of cypress oil, lemon, and mandarin oil, mix, add a tablespoon of any of the base oil and take a bath with the addition of this tool. Bath time - 15-20 minutes.
4. Relaxing bath: 2 - 6 drops diluted in kefir, yogurt, milk or cream, add in a bath of slightly warmer water. Time of procedure - 10-15 minutes.
5. Massage: in 20g.of the base oil or cream add 3 - 5 drops of cypress oil. As a basis we can take olive oil, soybean oil or peach.
6. Means for cleansing oily skin: Mix 4 drops of tangerine and cypress oils, add 3 drops of juniper oil and 20 ml of jojoba oil. Cleanser ready.
7. Steam bath to cleanse the pores of the skin: take a vessel with hot water, add 2-3 drops of cypress, fir or juniper oil, take a bath for 15 minutes, wash with cool water.
8. Tonic for oily skin: Mix equal parts of lemon oil, sandalwood, cypress and mint, add water. In one application typically takes 2 drops of each oil and 30 ml. of water. This composition is rubbed in facial skin. **Warning:** the peppermint oil – in some people it causes an allergic reaction, that's why pre-test for interaction with the oil.
9. Face cream: add oil at the rate of 4-5 drops per 20 g. of basic cream.
10. Shampoo: Mix 120 ml. of liquid soap with 60 ml of water, add 0.5 teaspoon of base oils (olive, avocado). Add 10 drops of cypress oil. All mix well, wash your hair. **Warning:** this tool is not for everyone, so it is best to prepare a small batch and test, and then decide - it's your or not.
11. Hair conditioner: Apply to brush one drop of oil, comb your hair in different directions.

12. Hair mask: make the mask before washing the head: 20ml base oil (olive, jojoba) are mixed with 10 drops of cypress oil, a little warm up on water bath and rub into the scalp and distribute through hair. Close the head with warm towel and leave for an hour.
13. Cypress oil for hands and nails: Apply a drop of oil on your hands, distribute evenly, capturing nails. This procedure will save your hands from the aging of skin, will give fortress to your nails.

Cedar oil: useful properties, treatment, use. Cedar oil in cosmetics, for face, hands, nails and hair.

Pine nut - the fruit of a cedar pine. This species are native to Japan, China, Mongolia, North Korea, North America and Russia, it is a evergreen tree that grows up to 40 meters high and up to 2 meters in diameter. Cedar can live up to 350 years, and some trees up to 800 years. Pine nut develops only in the upper part of the crown, and it has rich harvest once every 5 years, although the tree fruiting once every two years.

Cedar oil can be obtained by two ways: by cold and hot pressing. Oil cold "spin" is appreciated for its taste and healing properties. It has a great nutty flavor, amber color and it features a large protein and polyunsaturated fatty acids. As part of the protein are amino acids - arginine, which is essential for proper development of the growing organism (children, adolescents, pregnant women).

By processing the nuts is obtained by hot-pressing, technical oil, which is used in medicine, perfume industry, as well as in the production of paints and varnishes.

Useful properties of cedar oil

Oil of cedar nuts - a special oil, primarily, because of its medicinal properties, in the second, due to the fact that today there is no possibility to create an analogue of this oil by synthetic means, and thirdly, because it has no *contraindications for consumption.*

Cedar oil is easily absorbed by the child and adult body. It is rich in vitamins, minerals, trace elements and polyunsaturated fatty acids. Cedar oil is rich in vitamins of groups B and D, *normalizes the activity of the central nervous system and improves blood formation.* Its regular use can solve the problem of avitaminosis. According to the number of vitamin E per unit of weight of cedar oil, it exceeds olive and coconut oils. This refers to the active vitamin antioxidant group and reduces blood cholesterol. Furthermore, in cedar oil is very high content of vitamin F, three times higher than in the fish oil. This vitamin also has the ability to *lower cholesterol and strengthen immunity to respiratory disease.* In addition, vitamin F promotes lactation in nursing mothers, and prevents atherosclerosis.

Treatment with cedar oil

Laboratory studies confirmed the arising effect from the use of cedar oil in diseases such as:

1. SARS, influenza;
2. psoriasis;
3. gastric ulcer and duodenal ulcer;
4. hemorrhoids;
5. allergy;
6. atopic dermatitis;
7. skin diseases;
8. metabolic disease;
9. baldness.

Cedar oil has *healing properties, it accelerates epithelization of wounds, burns and frostbite.* It can have a *restorative effect, improve physical and mental performance, it also helps to cope with chronic fatigue syndrome, enhances immunity, improves vision and removes salt from the body of heavy metals, radionuclides and other toxins.*

The use of cedar oil

- Internal method of application: up to 3 times a day before eating, half a teaspoon each time. Usually the course lasts for 3 months under the scheme - 10 days of receiving to 5 days break. With cedar oil you can be refill vegetable salads, add to hot and cold snacks, so you will ensure the dish excellent taste characteristics, and for the body, healthy nutrients. The original cedar oil can be purchased at a price of 30 dollars per 0.5 liter. But beware of fakes and give preference to proven commercial organizations and well-established manufacturers.

Essential oil of mandarin: composition and properties. The use and treatment with mandarin oil. Essential oil of tangerine in cosmetology.

Essential oil of mandarin - orange liquid or dark orange, sometimes with reddish-yellow color with a very gentle, sweet, citrus aroma.

Homeland of the fruit is- south China and south Vietnam. It is an evergreen tree from the family Rutaceae, whose height is no more than 4 meters. It has a small shiny leaves, fragrant flowers and juicy fruits. It name the tree has received because of its exquisite and delicious fruit served on a table only for Mandarins - the rulers of the country. In Europe, the mandarins have appeared only in the early 19th century. Currently, they are quite common in Algeria, Spain, France, Indochina.

Since ancient times, tangerine peel was used in medicine of Eastern countries to improve digestion and appetite, to relieve inflammation in the throat and bronchi, to mitigate the suffocating cough.

Today, due to its composition and useful properties of mandarin, essential oil is widely used not only in medicine, but also cosmetics.

The composition of essential oils of mandarin

Tangerine oil is obtained by cold pressing, pressing of the fresh peel of ripe fruits. It is composed of limonene, myrcene, caryophyllene and pinene, camphene and contain: linalool, geraniol, nerol and other components allowing use of oil not only in medicine and cosmetics, but also as a food additive and perfume.

Properties of mandarin oil

Essential oil of mandarin - a pledge of beauty in the sun during the winter deficit. No wonder that in America it is called "solar heart." It helps *absorb vitamins, increases the body's own protective properties, enhances appetite, improves digestion, cleanses the body from toxins.* In addition, it is subject to stimulate the liver to regulate metabolic processes and the breakdown of fats, not to mention the secretion of bile. Tangerine oil is characterized by a*ntiseptic, antispasmodic, anti-scorbutic, anti-fungal and anti-inflammatory action.* It significantly optimizes the *exchange of blood, eliminates inflammation and bleeding gums.* In addition, is very effective in the *fight against excess weight, because it prevents the accumulation of kilograms, it displays the excess liquid and actively counteracts cellulite.*

An important property of tangerine oil is its *softness*. It is widely known for its gentle action, **because even pregnant women, children and those who are prone to allergies, may not be afraid to use it.**

It is simply irreplaceable for *irritability, fatigue, overexertion.* Its soothing effect has a beneficial effect on adult and *children's sleep and behavior.* Tangerine oil helps to recover faster after an illness or a mental crisis. By stimulating the nervous system, it eliminates *the feeling of fear.*

The use of essential oils of mandarin
Treatment with tangerine oil:

1. For therapeutic purposes, tangerine essential oil is widely used in various fields. Depending on the disease, it can be used by inhalation, rubbing, bath, internal use, as well as spraying for the rooms. Inhalation: *for colds, coughs, upper respiratory tract infections, use for inhalation a few drops of mandarin oil.* Do not forget about the deep of breathing and the time of inhalation (about 10 minutes).
2. Oil burner: for fatigue, overexertion, insomnia, irritability, light the aroma lamp with 3-5 drops of mandarin oil.
3. Aroma bath: an excellent tool in the fight against excess weight, cellulite, swelling, stretch marks, slag in the body, as well as for a charge of vivacity and energy. For the bath is enough to take 3-5 drops of oil.
4. Aroma medallion: 2-3 drops of essential oils of mandarin, hidden in aroma medallion, gives energy, joy and commitment for the whole working day.
5. Aromatization for liquid food: you can add 1-2 drops of oil in a plate of food or a glass of drink.
6. Massage: take 6-7 drops of mandarin oil during the massage, will have a tonic and restorative effect for the whole body.
7. Application to the gums: helps reduce inflammation, bleeding gums. Just add 5 drops of mandarin oil in 10 g of rosehip oil or wheat germ.
8. For rinse: a glass of warm water with 2-3 drops of oil is indispensable for sore throat, as well as for diseases of the oral cavity.
9. Internal use: for irritability, abdominal pain, difficulty swallowing, take a teaspoon of honey with the addition of 2-3 drops of oil. As an option - with herbal tea. Stimulation of gastric and intestinal activity is granted. It also cleansing of the body. To do this, you must have a drink in the morning on an empty stomach, take 3 drops of oil with water and honey; in the afternoon take 4 drops of mandarin oil and add half a teaspoon of honey and a cup of acid water. During

the day, you can not drink tea and coffee, and you must have an easy dinner. This technique of using essential oils of mandarin can quickly cleanse the body and, therefore, help in reducing weight.

Essential oil of tangerine in cosmetology

Essential oil of mandarin - unique cosmetic means capable of amazing tone and refresh *tired, flabby skin.* Moreover, it has *the strength to align the relief epidermis.* Most often it is used with a view to restore *skin elasticity and firmness, remove cellulite, eliminate pigmentation.* Tangerine oil fine improves skin tone and condition.

Note! Do not use mandarin oil on the skin before going out, as the sunlight falling on the oil can cause burns. You also can not use oil in case of intolerance.

- Enrichment of cosmetics: it is necessary to put 5-8 drops of oil in the 15g. base (during cleansing, toning, moisturizing, nourishing the skin).
- Massage: only 5-7 drops of mandarin oil, applied to the 15 ml of base oil, can quickly and effectively help the sagging skin to get rid of cellulite and stretch marks. *A great recipe for preventing the appearance of stretch marks in pregnant women for the skin of the abdomen:* take 5 drops of mandarin oil, 5 drops of neroli and lavender- 10 drops per 10 ml of wheat germ oil and 40 ml of almond oil. With resulting mixture make massage on affected areas at least 1-3 times a day.

Essential oil of mandarin - one of the most valuable and the best gifts that nature has given to us. It variety of useful properties and applications allow you to easily and quickly get the desired therapeutic and cosmetic effect, even at home.

Sea buckthorn oil: A useful composition, the use and treatment with sea buckthorn oil. Recipes with sea buckthorn.

Sea buckthorn - a plant that is widely known for its healing properties. People treated with it since ancient times, using both external and internal remedy for many diseases and problems.

Sea buckthorn oil and the juice are taken if needed to recover from a *serious illness; with juice of berries and leaf decoction you may wash the wound; oil is used for burns, diseases of the gastrointestinal tract, female diseases, sore throat, joint pain, sinusitis, atherosclerosis, diseases of the skin and hair.* The oil of this plant have different magical, healing properties - *soothes pain, reduces inflammation, stimulates the healing of wounds and ulcers, protects against infections.*

A useful composition of sea buckthorn oil

Fruits of sea buckthorn oil may contain from 5 to 10% of oil. This oil has a distinctive, bright orange color - due to the high content of *carotenoids*. The chemical composition of sea buckthorn oil is very rich: it contains a lot of biologically active substances - tocopherols, organic acids, phospholipids, phytosterols, vitamins, many minerals and amino acids, palmitic acid, palmitoleic acid, most of the vitamins A, E and C.

Treatment with sea buckthorn oil. Recipes with Sea Buckthorn

Sea buckthorn oil is used in medicine or cosmetics - the official medicine uses it to treat various diseases. On the basis of sea buckthorn oil are made a lot of medications given to patients to treat and prevent many health problems.

Sea buckthorn oil treats *abscesses and boils, fistulas, ulcers, trauma and inflammation of the mucous membranes of the tumor.* In cancer of the esophagus is prescribed during radiotherapy, and *even for 2-3 weeks after the end of treatment - 0.5 tsp./ 3 times a day.*

Sea-buckthorn oil stimulates sexual function, has a favorable effect on the thyroid gland; *it is useful in the treatment of atherosclerosis, improves heart, blood vessels makes elastic*; It supports normal cholesterol level, participates in the metabolism of proteins, prevents fatty liver; can output salts of heavy metals, kill disease-causing by germs, protects liver. If with sea buckthorn oil you will lubricate the throat and nasal passages than tonsillitis, pharyngitis, rhinitis, tonsillitis, are cured faster. Lubricating the joints daily can relieve gout and rheumatism.

Affected tissues and trophic ulcers heal faster, if they are treated with buckthorn oil - a complex of substances contained in it, has a strong regenerating properties. Burns moderate are healed almost without a trace; with sea buckthorn oil you can treat even sunburn.

Most often, sea buckthorn oil used to treat diseases of the gastrointestinal tract: *gastritis, colitis, gastric ulcer and duodenal ulcer.* Increased acidity of the oil contributes to its reduction, heals ulcers and scars.

In gastric ulcer sea buckthorn oil must be taken 2-3 times a day, half an hour before meals-1 tsp.. *However, in pancreatitis, acute cholecystitis and other diseases of the pancreas the sea buckthorn oil is contraindicated.* In the propensity to diarrhea and indigestion, it is also not recommended – or it should be used with caution.

- Candles with sea buckthorn oil, *well heal anal fissures, ulcers and inflammation of the rectum.*
- In dental practice sea buckthorn oil is used in treatment of *periodontitis* - an inflammation of the tissues surrounding the roots of teeth; *stomatitis and pulpitis* - inflammation of dental pulp.
- Sea buckthorn oil helps our eyes - this is confirmed by many ophthalmologists. With its help you may treat *corneal defects and injuries, conjunctivitis, ulcer, keratitis; severe eye burns, including chemical; Trachoma - chronic infectious eye disease; radiation damage.*

Most women know that sea buckthorn oil has long been used in gynecology, and gives an excellent effect in the treatment of many diseases.

- In inflammation of the mucous membrane of the vagina and the cervix, sea buckthorn oil is introduced into the vagina with a cotton swab. The same treatment is prescribed for endocervicites - more extensive inflammation of the mucous membrane of the cervix and cervical canal. The course usually last up to 2 weeks.
- In cervical erosion sea buckthorn oil - it is administered, by many gynecologists. 1-2 weeks it must be inserted into the vagina wit a soaked swab, tightly pressing it to the cervix - the oil on the swab should be about 5-10 ml, and leave it for at least 12 hours. After 2 months, you can repeat the procedure.
- Buckthorn oil, has ability to soften the skin, making it more elastic and protect against free radicals, it is widely used in cosmetology. On the basis of this oil are produced creams, masks, balms, shampoos, toothpaste, lipstick, cosmetic creams, etc.
- Sea buckthorn oil fading and wrinkled skin: improves its tone, increases firmness and elasticity, smoothes shallow wrinkles. If you have dry skin on the face, apply this oil – it will softens, moisturizes and nourishes dry skin, prevents its aging and the appearance of wrinkles.
- Brown spots and freckles, too, can be removed or lighten with the help of sea buckthorn oil. It treat damaged skin, acne, eczema, dermatitis, pyoderma, erythematosus, lichen, and many skin diseases.
- Sea-buckthorn oil is perfectly for cares of lips and skin around the eyes, nourishes and strengthens lashes.

For cleaning do not use undiluted oil – with clean oil are lubricated only damaged or diseased skin at the affected sites. In general, for cosmetic purposes is used sea buckthorn oil, obtainable by the process of cold pressing.

- You can add it to your daily face cream: taking on the palm a portion of the cream, add to it a few drops of oil, mix and then apply on face.

Face masks with sea buckthorn oil

With sea buckthorn oil, you can make homemade masks for the face - a lot of them. Here are some of them:

- For dry, aging skin. Mix 1 tsp. of oil and fresh sea buckthorn juice with a raw egg yolk and apply the mixture on your face for 15-20 minutes; wash off the mask with warm water lightly. If there is no juice of sea buckthorn berries, then instead, you can take the apple, orange, grape, peach or apricot - certainly fresh.
- For aging and dull skin – apply 2 times a week. Raw egg yolk mix with 1 tsp. of sea buckthorn oil and add 0.5 l. of yellow powder of cosmetic clay. Stir well to avoid lumps left, and apply on face for 15 minutes. Rinse first with warm water, then cool. This mask tightens the skin, making it more elastic and fresh.
- Mask of sea buckthorn oil and cottage cheese is more suitable for dry skin, but it can also be used for aging. Take 3 tablespoons of warm milk, dissolve in it 1 tsp. of honey, then add 1 tablespoon of fat cottage cheese and 1 tsp. of sea buckthorn oil, and triturate everything. Put mixture on the face, and after 15 minutes with wet fingers gently roll up like in the application of scrubs. Residues can be removed with warm water.
- For the treatment of hair - it can be prepared at home. Chopped burdock root - 3 tsp., pour 1.5 cups of water, put on fire, bring to a boil; cook for 15 minutes on low heat. The resulting broth drain, add 5 tablespoons of sea buckthorn oil and beat. This cream is suitable for fine and dry hair. If you regularly rub it into the scalp, the hair will become healthy shine, become stronger and stronger.

How to cook sea buckthorn oil

Sea buckthorn oil can be made at home, by a fairly simple way. Get fresh berries , wash and dry, spread out on a cloth or paper. You will need to squeeze the juice with the help of the press, pour it into the jar and put in a dark place for 2 weeks.

On the surface layer of oil will form juice - it is necessary to collect, via pipette or conventional spoons and pasteurize it. Fruits left in the bank, can also be used: it is good for homemade jellies and beverages.

Perhaps from all the medicinal plants, buckthorn is among the most popular, including the official medicine. **However, any treatment of folk remedies, including sea buckthorn oil, should start after the recommendations of experts.**

Sage essential oil: structure, properties, application to hair, skin, hands and nails. Treatment with oil of sage.

About the medicinal properties of sage is known since the time of the first dynasties of Egyptian pharaohs. Even in ancient times with the help of sage treat *infertility*, and in the Middle Ages it was used to protect against the plague. Today, Sage is valued in cooking, cosmetics and medicine. Confectioners are very well aware of this spice that is able to give any dish a bitter and unique taste. In the medicinal and cosmetic purposes are used drugs from the flowers and leaves of the plant, as well as the essential oil of sage.

Sage has *antiseptic, anti-inflammatory, antispasmodic, expectorant properties, it promotes healing of wounds, helps with any bleeding, anti-inflammatory action, and therefore it is used in all diseases of the body, which are accompanied by inflammation.*

The composition of the essential oil of sage

The composition of the oil of sage is not fully known. Today there are more than 20 substances included in the oils of sage, which are necessary to the human body and can have a beneficial effect on him. It includes salve, D-a-pinene, peel, D-camphor, terpenoids, cineole, a- and b-thujone, a variety of alkaloids and flavonoids, linoleic acid glycerides. They make from sage essential oil a strong pale yellow, transparent liquid having bluff but pleasant and original flavor.

The most potent medically sage substance - it *Salvini* - quite a powerful *natural antibiotic*. This concentrated blend of organic acids, which is quite effective at on a range of bacteria and microorganisms. For example, it has been demonstrated that 5 minutes of rinsing with sage oil the mouth or throat is enough for bacteria to be killed, as well as restore the natural microflora.

Treatment with sage oil

Sage oil has a regulating effect on *hormone levels, also has anti-inflammatory effect, leading to tone the uterus.* It is used for *painful menstruation and heavy bleeding women.* By the way, heavy bleeding at all - it is also a testimony to the use of sage oil.

As an *astringent, expectorant and anti-inflammatory* oil of sage is used for any respiratory diseases, such as tuberculosis, bronchial asthma, chronic and acute bronchitis, and various respiratory diseases. It is also known that is effective use of sage oil in *dermatology,* diseases of the *musculoskeletal system,* various diseases of the *gastrointestinal tract, circulatory system,* etc.

For topical use: sage oil is indispensable for wounds and sores as a wound healing and antiseptic. Rinse the mouth with sage oil in *gingivitis, stomatitis and angina, especially with complications, helps eliminate bad breath.*

Essential oil of sage for hair

In cosmetic essential oils are widely used, and their cosmetic properties are also well known. Sage oil - is no exception. It has long been known the tonic effect on hair of oil of sage. Thanks to antiseptic properties of sage oil on the scalp it may cure *dandruff, seborrhea, and various skin diseases of the head and even alopecia.*

It helps sage quite effectively and with hair loss, and a variety of masks for the hair oil of sage in combination with other essential oils and extracts, can achieve excellent results in hair strengthening. It is very useful to make a mask of essential oils before washing the head. Mask are slightly warmed in a water bath and gently massaged, are rubbed into the skin of the head with fingers. After that the hair should be wrapped in plastic wrap or a towel. The mask rests on the head for about an hour. The course of treatment - 20 days daily. These procedures will help to make your hair silky and shiny.

Sage oil for the skin

Due to its antiseptic and wound-healing properties, sage oil is very effective in various skin diseases. For medical purposes sage oil is used topically for various inflammations of the skin, such as pustular. Also it is used for *burns, cuts and abrasions, bruises.* In addition, thanks to its distinctive flavor, sage oil *repels mosquitoes and can be used as a means for mosquito.*

Most athletes use sage oil is to heat up the muscles before exercise.

In cosmetology oil of sage is used in the treatment of *acne eruptions on the skin.* It is the tonic effect on the skin, sage oil has *regenerative and anti-allergenic properties, improves blood circulation.*

Sage oil for hands and nails

Curative effect of sage oil on hands and nails are also long been known. Your skin is very delicate and the most exposed to influences from the outside, and therefore quickly grows coarse, it starts to peel off. Also, sage oil is effective in treating the layers of nails.

Formulations with sage oil *nourish the skin, making it soft and smooth, provide nail care, prevent their separation, strengthen them*. Especially effective essential oil of sage is when your skin is dry and damaged.

Peppermint essential oil: the use, composition and properties. The use of essential oil of mint: recipes from peppermint oil.

Scents that produces mint has on the human body a physical, mental and emotional impact. The molecules from what is composed the essential oil of peppermint, likely to affect the human nervous system, thus correcting the emotional state and physical activity. Peppermint essential oil the aroma able *to tone the tired body, rejuvenate and de-stress*. The smell of peppermint has a very favorable effect at the moment when you need to cheer up, buck up and keep a job or some other important work. Excellent effect has on the nervous system, a bright and fresh aroma is able to magically awaken anyone.

Interesting peppermint essential oil effect is that it *increases the mental activity of the fair sex*. The smell of peppermint increases *confidence, removes tension and stiffness, refreshing and truly invigorating*.

Not less effective essential oil of mint acts for *colds, perfectly kills viruses and bacteria, can reduce body temperature*.

Essential peppermint oil fight with *loss of voice and mild hoarseness*, gives soothing effect. Significantly improves *cerebral blood flow, affects the blood vessels, as an antispasmodic agent*.

Peppermint essential oil can quickly remove almost any *kind of pain, like headaches and menstrual, muscular*. In a toothache at the time the oil is able to numb the pain, in addition, mint is well eliminates *bad breath*.

For people suffering from seasickness peppermint oil is salvage, it eliminates *vomiting, dizziness and nausea.*

The peppermint oil is part of some well-known cardiac drugs others drugs.

The composition of the essential oil of peppermint

Is obtained the essential oil of peppermint from the flowering tops of the plant, as well as the first leaves. If we talk about the chemical composition of essential oil of mint, it is this: carvacrol, menthol, pinene, terpinene, menthyl acetate, cineole, phellandrene, limonene, thymol, neomenthol.

Peppermint essential oil is the lightest of all the oils because it containing menthol, it has been successfully used in cosmetology, and is suitable for all skin types.

The use of oil for oily skin provides a narrowing of pores, adjustment of the sebaceous glands. In dry skin peppermint oil helps *to retain moisture.* In addition, mint removes *signs of fatigue,* the use of this oil is quite noticeable in that people that did not sleep all night. Best suited specifically for *oily skin, eliminating inflammation, acne, bacterial dermatitis.* Peppermint essential oil can improve the skin in the first signs of *eczema.*

The use of essential oil of mint: recipes from peppermint oil

1. Aroma lamps about 4-6 drops: Inhalation of fine fragrance activates brain activity. Refreshing and invigorating smell. It eliminates from air the bacteria, which is important during the various epidemics.
2. With the help of peppermint oil can be carried out warm inhalation. To do this: add about 2-4 drops of oil. Treatment time must not exceed 5 minutes.
3. With peppermint oil you can take hot baths, for this: add to the water 2-6 drops of oil.
4. Massage and compresses with peppermint oils as well are very useful for the organism. In pure form, applying oil to the skin is not necessary.
5. Oil may be added to the core cream for cosmetic purposes, approximately 6 drops per 15 grams of the cream.

It is recommended to mix peppermint oil with a vegetable ones and used in the following cases:

1. In colds: rub the chest with oil;
2. In skin itch: rub the problem areas;
3. In the pain in the muscles or joints: rub the problem area;
4. In rheumatoid arthritis;

5. If 5-7 drops of peppermint oil are added to 10 ml. of alcohol, you get an excellent alcohol solution, which is used for the sauna.
6. Undiluted peppermint oil 1-2 droplets are applied on the tooth, as an analgesic.
7. For protection against insects, drip a few drops of any area of the skin;
8. In aroma medallion: use 2 drops;
9. Inside mint oil can be used to treat heartburn, but do so with extreme caution, adding 2 drops in a tablespoon of yogurt.
10. You can add 1 drop of oil to jam and drink tea or yogurt, juice with it.

Add 6-8 drops of peppermint essential oil in your tea, you will get incredibly delicious and aromatic tea. It has a *carminative, diaphoretic, antispasmodic, antiseptic, analgesic effect*. Good effect have on the stomach, *liquefies phlegm, increases mental activity*. You can use it as a tea in elevated temperature, general loss of strength.

Apart from the fact that the essential oil of mint have a superb pharmaceuticals and cosmetics properties, it is used successfully in culinary. Besides, that the smell of mint is categorically not tolerate by insects, so it can be an excellent repellent. And if you put it in aroma lamps, mint oil, or just sprinkle it around, where are *rodents and cockroaches*, very soon pests run away from this place and will not come back. And if you mix the mint with some other scented oil, such as eucalyptus, the effect will be even brighter, and rodents will simply leave, not die, as when using pesticides.

For pets and children it is absolutely harmless.

Contraindications for peppermint oil

Strongly is not recommended to apply peppermint oil on the skin of children younger than seven years. You can not use this oil for bronchitis, since it can reduce, if not cancel the effect of medicines.

Do not use peppermint oil in the evening because it may cause sleep disturbance, oil invigorates and sleep will be difficult.

It not recommended to use the oil throughout pregnancy and also during lactation. It is necessary to avoid the application of peppermint oil to the eye area. In addition, peppermint essential oil can cause allergies. Therefore, before the first application you must test for individual tolerance.

Grape seed oil: Structure, properties and applications. Grape seed oil for face and body.

From long ago have been known for its healing properties and it is used in medicine and cosmetics for centuries. It is called the "youth hormone" for its high content of *vitamin R*. This vitamin complex is essential for the human connections that prevent capillary fragility.

Grape seed oil has a relatively light texture, which is why it is successfully used for oily and combination skin. Grape seed oil is quickly absorbed and helps to improve the work of the sebaceous glands. In addition, *fine tightens pores, giving the skin a healthy and well-groomed appearance.*

Because of *procyanidins*, an antioxidant that is found in grape seed oil, with the systematic application, helps rid the body from aggressive radicals. This promotes natural improve in overall health and increase immunity.

Grape seed oil is rich in a variety of vitamins and microelements that are used in cosmetology. A special place among them has, vitamin E, known for its medicinal and nutritional properties.

The use of grape seed oil

In cosmetology grape seed oil is used for a variety of procedures due to its reducing effect. The application of oil on the delicate breast skin, protects it from *premature aging*. Regenerating and moisturizing oil property, helps in the process of *losing weight and to maintain the elasticity of the body.*

For therapeutic purposes: grape seed oil is rubbed into the scalp to stimulate *hair growth, strengthen hair against breakage and make them shine.* In *rosacea* treatments apply this oil, because it not only strengthens blood vessels, but also makes them more flexible. Also, the oil has been successfully used to improve the appearance of nails and softening the skin. Big content of linolenic acid in the grape seed oil restores normal skin work. *Regeneration* ability of oil, help quickly and without a trace to solve the problem of *acne*, minimize the effects *of burns and wounds*, as well as restore the skin after the negative impact with the external environment.

The light texture of the oil you can use it as a means to *care for hands, soften cuticles and strengthen nails.*

Grapeseed oil - is the perfect vitamin complex, which affects the entire body, from the skin enriching micronutrients, and ending with the treatment of various diseases, in combination with other drugs. It is used to *lower cholesterol*, for the treatment of *cellulite and vascular diseases*, while providing *anti-inflammatory and tonic effect.*

Oxidants, are part of the grape seed oil that slow down the *natural aging process*, and vitamin composition of the oil has an even more pronounced effect in the fight against aging. Vitamin E, which is part of the oil, prevent *cardiovascular and oncological diseases* caused by blockage of blood vessels and high blood cholesterol.

The composition of grape seed oil
Is a storehouse of useful trace elements and compounds. Among them are: *Vitamin E* that moisturizes and nourishes the skin; *linoleic acid-* accelerates tissue regeneration process; *tannins-* with draining effect. In addition, *chlorophyll* contained in this oil, accelerates metabolism.

The cosmetic use of grape seed oil, as a separate ingredient, or as a supplement in the various cosmetic preparations.
Because of it properties is well absorbed and penetrate deep into the tissue; it is used as a basis for the creation of masks, tonics, essential cosmetic formulations. The most commonly, oil is used in the composition of moisturizing lipsticks, regenerating creams and shampoos for damaged and dull hairs. Combined with seed oils of lemon, avocado, ylang-ylang and jojoba oil it is used for *therapeutic anti-cellulite massage.*

Grape seed oil for face and body
- Massage: rub grape seed oil in your hands. With easy movement, rub oil into the skin until completely absorbed.
- Anti-cellulite massage: base - grape seed oil, mix with essential oils: jojoba - 4 drops, almond - 10 drops. Massage should be done on a heated body after a sauna bath or after a warm bath. After the massage, you need to lie down for 15-30 minutes.
- Wraps: grape seed oil is uniformly applied to the problem area, gently rub in the skin and cover with cling film. It is necessary to wear warm pants or lie down under a blanket for warming and improving the effect. Duration of procedure - 30 minutes, after which you need a gauze pad soaked in warm water to wipe the oil residue.
- Packs for oily skin: grape seed oil as a basis, add a few drops of oil of ylang-ylang, chamomile and lemon, then a soak in a cotton swab and apply to problem skin- 2-3 times a day.

- Face masks: grape seed oil, almond oil, take them in equal proportions, moisten a pad in this mixture and apply it on your face for 15-25 minutes. After the procedure, cleane with warm water.
- Bath: a tablespoon of grape oil is dissolved in 3 tablespoons of honey, add in a warm bath. Bath time: from 15 to 20 minutes. During the reception of such treatment, bath soaps and gels are not used. After the 30 minutes, your blood circulation will be improved .

If you have an allergy to grape seed oil, then limit yourself to its application.

Wheat germ oil: properties and benefits. Wheat germ oil for face, hair (mask) and stretch marks.

Since ancient times people knew that from small grains of wheat germ can be obtained a special oil. Wheat germ oil - a true gift of nature, filled with lots of vitamins and minerals, numerous active ingredients that make up the embryo, are also found in the oil. This valuable product is used not only in the food industry as for food additives, but also in various fields of medicine for the treatment of many diseases. And now, more and more popularity is gaining the use of essential oils of wheat germ in many areas of cosmetology. The oil obtained from wheat germ, is one of the richest on the content of vitamin E in it, which is simply necessary for the maintenance and extension of our skin youthful. We can say that it includes also other, not less important vitamins - A, B, D, PP, as many polyunsaturated acids, lecithin, and other elements that can affect the skin condition of people.

Properties and benefits of wheat germ oil

The use of wheat germ oil is very effective in stimulating the processes of *renewal and rejuvenation of cells*, while it helps significantly to improve the skin's health and appearance. **Also, the product has no contraindications and can be used for all types of skin - and dry, and more fat.**

Wheat germ oil has an excellent effect for *softening and moisturizing and nourishing the skin with all the necessary micro-elements*, and that is what makes it so comfortable to use for care of dried, rough or flaky skin.

High efficiency oil from wheat germ have found the application in the care of the *old and aging skin*, which already beginning to lose its natural properties - the freshness, elasticity. The tool helps a lot to *rejuvenate the skin, significantly tighten oval face, perfectly smooth all kinds of wrinkles, increases and strengthens the skin tone* layers. Oil, pressed from young sprouts of wheat, has great *cleansing effect*, and good cleans the skin and its pores from all kinds of pollution, which is simply impossible to avoid. And the oil's ability to *eliminate all kinds of harmful and dangerous toxins, various harmful substances* from the skin, simply excels in cosmetics.

Important is the *active anti-inflammatory action*, which can be seen in contact with the inflamed skin oils. All this makes it very effectively and successfully used in the care of oily and contaminated skin. The oil of wheat germs, very effectively combats all kinds of skin problems such as *acne, pustular lesions, and other kinds of inflammation that are harmful*, not only to deterioration the appearance of the skin, but also to lead to other, more serious illness.

Everything contained in the oil, have a very strong *healing effect on burns, cuts, bruises, and many, many other skin lesions, and can help in diseases such as all kinds of dermatitis, eczema, neurodermatitis*, that have significant risk to the health of human skin.

The remarkable *toning, refreshing and smoothing of skin, improve complexion* - all these activities are very active and efficacious when you use wheat oil, because it is a completely natural product, which in no way can worsen the condition of your health, but on the contrary, *will help you deal with your skin problems* .

In addition, oil obtained from wheat germ, can be used for *rejuvenation* of the skin around the eye area, as well as in the care of the lips, cracked or chapped lips, or for the treatment of cracks in the corners of the mouth.

The use of wheat germ oil in cosmetics
The main methods of using wheat germ oil in cosmetics for face.

Due to the fact that the oil obtained from wheat germ is very dense in structure, its use for cosmetic purposes in a pure form is not desirable because of its relative "hardness". The main method of its use - *mixing it with other, lighter oils of vegetable origin.*

Of course, is possible to use wheat germ oil in its pure form, not diluted with other substances, but it is recommended to do so only on small areas of the skin. For example, a small amount of it can lubricate the skin places most prone to peeling or the hardened areas. You can also apply wheat germ oil to the most problematic areas - inflammation, irritation, all kinds of itch, acne, ulcers, burns, wounds. Is acceptable use of wheat germ oil in its pure form *for the wrinkles on the face*, for example, on the forehead , eye corners. But for use on areas of skin under the eyes oil *is not suitable* because of its severity, the skin around the eyes is particularly thin. For such applications it is recommended to dilute it at a ratio of one to three with rosehip oil or with any other essential oil. Such a mixture can be used daily for the treatment of *aging*.

Wheat germ oil for the face

Masks based on wheat germ oil:

1. Mask for sagging, wrinkles, aging skin: Take 3 teaspoons of wheat germ oil and add 1 drop of peppermint oil, orange and sandalwood. Apply the resulting mass on a paper towel and put it on the face, but no more than 20 minutes. Do not rinse the mask. Its remnants soak into the skin.
2. Mask for oily skin covered with acne: 3 teaspoons of wheat germ oil, 2 drops of lavender oil, cedar or clove. Apply on the face as well as in the above mask.
3. Mask to remove freckles and spots on the skin: 3 teaspoons of wheat germ oil, 1 drop of lemon oil, bergamot and juniper. Apply the mixture on the napkin, the mask is applied to the skin 2 times a day for 20-30 minutes. The same can be done using only a wheat germ oil.
4. To get rid of wrinkles around the eyes, can help the following composition: 3 teaspoons of wheat germ oil, 1 drop of sandalwood and neroli or 2 drops of rose oil. Apply with light circular movements of the fingers on the skin surface of the eyelids and around the mouth until the oil is completely absorbed.
5. The mask for dry and problem skin of the face and lips: use wheat germ oil without impurities, or add 1 drop of lemon balm and rose oil. Treat the skin 2-3 times a day.

Wheat germ oil for hair

1. Mask for strengthening hair: It is recommended to apply only wheat germ oil on the scalp or use a mixture of jojoba oil in the ratio 1: 1.
2. Additionally, wheat germ oil can be mixed with 2 drops of pine oil, cedar, eucalyptus, ginger or orange oil and thyme. The resulting mixture is applied to the hair roots. Apply this mask to 20 minutes before washing the head.

For the prevention of, and to reduce stretch marks is indispensable wheat germ oil. It is soaking into scar tissue, smoothes from the inside, improving cell regeneration, and thus under constant procedures reduces the size and color of the stretch marks. Even if there is no stretch at this point, the daily rubbing with a light massage moves, makes the skin supple and prevents it to deform at different factors.

Prevention and treatment of diseases with wheat germ oil

Wheat germ oil is used for the prevention and treatment of various diseases, and as a food additive. Here are some of the ways to use wheat germ oil into the treatment of various diseases and the prevention of changes associated with aging.

1. To prevent diseases like gastritis and gastric ulcer: take one month/ one teaspoon of wheat germ oil, 1-2 times a day.
2. For the prevention of gastritis, colitis and ulcers, 2 hours after dinner drink a teaspoon of wheat germ oil.

Children aged 6 to 15 years, pregnant and lactating women, it is desirable to take 2-3 times a day a half of teaspoon. The duration of prophylactic treatment - at least 2 weeks.

Contraindications to the use of wheat oil

People suffering from diseases such as gallstone or kidney stone, is not desirable to use wheat germ oil.

The conditions of storage of wheat germ oil

Wheat germ oil can be stored up to 10 - 12 months, but only in the dark and tightly closed containers, at a temperature not higher than + 15C. After opening the jars with oil, it is stored in the refrigerator.

Grapefruit essential oil: composition and use. Grapefruit oil in cosmetology and facial hair. Indications and contraindications of grapefruit oil.

Many people do not realize what important a role in our lives play odors. But those who are aware of their magical powers, can not pass aromatherapy. One of the most popular is grapefruit essential oil.

Imagine a ten-meter tree with smooth, like a glossy photo paper, leaves. In the spring it is covered with white flowers, which will eventually turn into a yellow-orange fruit with a diameter of about fifteen centimeters. Grapefruit trees are the result of crossbreeding a pomelo and orange.

The composition and the use of essential oil of grapefruit

Grapefruit essential oil is not less popular than it fruits. This oil have a transparent yellow color, but may have a green tint. The process of oil production of grapefruit is no different from the manufacture of other essential compounds of citrus fruits. Each fruit peel is separated from the pulp, and by means of the press, but without the use of heat treatment, the oil is extruded. With worse quality is considered to be oil, which is obtained from the juice production residues (peel and pulp) and, if essential oil are produced by distillation of the initial product. Basically, grapefruit oil is produced in Israel, Brazil and the United States of America.

Experts identified a number of basic properties of essential oil of grapefruit. Firstly, it serves as a *diuretic*, secondly, has a *tonic and stimulating* effect, acts as an *antidepressant*, and thirdly, an excellent *antiseptic.*

Ways to use essential oils in aromatherapy are a lot. Let us dwell only on the most popular. If you feel too complex for, intolerant even to entourage, then you should try aroma cocktail . In the aromatic bulb is added one drop of essential oil of ylang-ylang, frankincense and grapefruit, as well as two drops of mandarin oil. This composition will *calm nerves, give courage, you will be kind and tolerant.* In addition, the elegant scent of grapefruit essential oil can relieve some people from complacency, and to the other will give confidence, helping to find common ground, even with strangers.

Grapefruit essential oil in cosmetics

Grapefruit facial hair oil:

If you want to increase the effectiveness of your cream, you can enrich them with various essential oils. For example, for oily skin will fit mixture of two drops of bergamot, lemon balm, and one drop of grapefruit. All this add to 10 milliliters of any neutral cream. If the skin pores are seen, in the cream is poured one drop of lemon, chamomile and grapefruit oil. If so, you want to give your skin tone, for example, after a hard day, before the party, then you can add in the cream: 3 drops of grapefruit oil, patchouli and ylang-ylang oils by two drops.

For many people, the first spring sun is inextricably linked with the appearance of irregular skin pigmentation including freckles. Massage mixture based on thirty milliliters of almond oil with grapefruit and rosewood oils (three drops each) and four drops of ginger, will lighten skin.

Experts recommend from time to time to pamper your face with steam baths. Make them as possible. At half-liter of water, add a drop of lemon balm, bergamot and grapefruit twice as much oil. This recipe is ideal for people who have oily skin. If you used to do face masks, do not deny yourself the pleasure to try this recipe for oily skin, prone to fat. To four parts of honey add one part of alcohol with one part of boiled water. Then you should add aromatic essential oils of grapefruit and tea tree (two drops). Before you can use the mask, you should be prepared using a hot compress that should be kept on the face for at least three minutes. The mask should not be left for more than a third of an hour. *The skin becomes firmer, the complexion improves.*

If you are *prone to depression,* then allow yourself ten or fifteen minutes, soak in a warm bath, in which add four drops of bergamot and grapefruit. It will help to cheer up a mixture of grapefruit and rosemary essential oils that are also diluted in warm water. And in the fight against *cellulite,* can help the essential oils of anise, vetiver, mint (one drop) and grapefruit (4 drops). All this are mixed with one hundred grams of sea salt and rub into the skin on problem areas.

- Hairs look greasy often within a few hours after washing. With this, you can deal effectively. In every 10 milliliters of shampoo, add three or four drops of essential oil of grapefruit.

The essential oil of grapefruit - help in everyday life
Very popular the grapefruit essential oil can become for housewives, because it is not only for cosmetic purposes. If you want to quickly and effectively clean up the plate from coffee or milk, then in hot water add a few drops of essential oil of grapefruit.

Contraindications grapefruit oil
Before you can use the essential oil of grapefruit note that even it, has a number of contraindications. Firstly, individual allergic intolerance of organism. Second, it should not use an aromatic oil if the sun will be on as the grapefruit have marked phototoxicity property.

Lavender essential oil: structure, benefits, treatment with lavender oil. Lavender essential oil in cosmetology: for hands, nails, skin and hair.

Lavender - recognized the queen of fragrances. This plant is so universal, that is used in many household and industrial areas of our lives. For example, in cooking, cosmetics, perfumery, household chemicals in production and, of course, medicine. This alternative medicine has long known as the ancient divination tool, which, over the centuries of use, has not lost its relevance. Currently, *the most widely used essential oil is from lavender*. It is widely used in aromatherapy as an independent means, as a component or in combination with other aromatic oils.

The composition of the essential oil of lavender

Lavender essential oil is obtained by water-steam distillation of lavender species Lavandula officinalis. All parts of this plant contain essential oil, but its greatest amount are accumulated in inflorescences. Lavender essential oil - it is light, colorless liquid which in the main part consists from the complex alcohol esters of L-linalool and some acids - acetic, caproic, valeric and butyric. The essential oil of lavender emit substances such as geraniol, herniarin, lavandiol, coumarin, caryophyllene, borneol. And the flowers are rich in tannins, bitterness, and resins.

Properties and healing action of the essential oil of lavender

Lavender essential oil has a pronounced *anticonvulsant, sedative and diuretic* effects. Thanks to the excellent lymphatic drainage action, lavender essential oil improves *blood circulation, stimulates the cardiovascular system and cerebral blood flow.* Lavender essential oil is a strong *antiseptic, antibacterial and regenerating tool,* is therefore used for *rapid healing of wounds, destruction of pathogenic microbes, resorption of scars and skin seals.* Clinical data confirm *the strong soothing and toning properties of lavender oil.* The scent of lavender normalizes the function of the nervous system and is used for *insomnia, nervousness and nervous related diseases, general weakness, fatigue, loss of power.* Lavender oil is used for all types of effects on the body, both internal and external, through aroma lamps, aroma medallions , sprays, baths, inhalation, douches, compresses and direct application to the skin. **It should be remembered about the strong chemical properties of essential oils and not to exceed the recommended doses and direct contact of pure form or undiluted oils to the mucous membranes.**

Lavender oil has the ability *to mute too sharp, strong and unpleasant odors.* The cosmetic compositions of the essential oil of lavender is combined with the best-invigorating citrus flavors, rose and rosemary, pine oil, spicy carnation, patchouli, sage and nutmeg.

The use of lavender oil for medicinal purposes

Since ancient times, extracts and lavender flowers were used in the treatment of *cardiovascular, neurological and inflammatory disease*, but the pure form os essential oil of lavender is not recommended for taking in, as it can cause severe irritation of the gastric mucosa.

The most popular medicinal properties of essential oil of lavender is its *antiseptic, antibacterial and regenerative effect.*

For therapeutic purposes, lavender essential oil is widely used:

1. For total relaxation, relieve stress and calm the body's, for sleep will be sufficient to use aroma lamp in the room.
2. Oil burner inhalations are used to stimulate the central nervous system, heart and lower blood pressure.
3. Applications with cold or hot inhalation method with the addition of essential oil of lavender helps with expectorant and antimicrobial effect for respiratory diseases and bronchitis.
4. Warm compresses with the addition of 5-7 drops of pure lavender essential oil have antirheumatic and analgesic effect.
5. Cold compresses are useful in the solar and thermal burns, ulcers and purulent skin lesions: 1 drop of lavender essential oil to 10 drops of oil-base.
6. With aroma bath are achieved strong choleretic, diuretic and diaphoretic effect that contributes to the treatment of urolithiasis, pyelonephritis, neuralgia and other internal inflammatory disease. Just 5-7 drops of lavender essential oil are added to a bath, this will have a total relaxing and calming effect. Aroma baths also used to treat depression, neuralgia and migraines.
7. For the treatment of skin diseases such as eczema, dermatitis, vitiligo, mycosis, to achieve maximum therapeutic effect is applied acupressure using pure lavender oil or essential oil blends.
8. Point Aroma Massage for face will be useful in nasal congestion, headaches.
9. Lavender aromatherapy also help reduce pain during labor and strengthen labor.

The use of lavender oil in cosmetics

Unique cosmetic properties of lavender are expressed in its *disinfecting, anti-inflammatory and dries impact.* This is due to the fairly frequent use of lavender essential oil in the manufacture of cosmetics for oily and combination skin.

Lavender essential oil for skin, hair, hands, nails

Pure lavender essential oil has a unique wound-healing properties, due to which decreases the likelihood of post-inflammatory scarring.

The healing properties of lavender oil can also help to regulate the production of sebum, which prevents the formation of greasy and clogging pores, and the skin thus remains matte and silky.

The drugs with the addition of lavender essential oil - an excellent tool for damaged and weakened hair. With continued use of lavender, hair get healthy, shine and get vitality, significantly reduced breakage and hair loss.

Lavender oil is effective in the treatment of *dandruff and alopecia*, it is necessary to rub the prepared oil into the scalp before each wash.

With lavender oil is recommended to enrich the already finished cosmetic products. For example, a few drops of lavender essential oil added to the hand cream will quickly heal minor traumas, without leaving scars and seals.

To strengthen nails is useful to rub 1 drop of lavender oil in the nail, immediately after the manicure.

It should be noted that the essential oil of lavender is perfect for *flavoring, deodorization and disinfection*. But do not forget that lavender oil, like any other essential oil, has an individual intolerance, as well as a number of contraindications. **Do not use lavender essential oil during pregnancy. Exercise caution in diseases such as epilepsy, hypotension, bronchial asthma, and it is not necessary to apply oil to the skin with severe rash or allergic dermatitis.**

Lemon essential oil: structure, benefits, treatment of lemon oil. The use of essential oil of lemon in cosmetics for skin, hair and nails.

Lemon essential oil - light yellow or light-green liquid that have a typical bitter cold and the smell of fresh lemon.

Homeland of lemon - China, India and the tropical Pacific islands. This evergreen plant is no more than 5 meters in height, from the genus citrus, unknown in the wild-growing form. Already in ancient Egypt, people used lemon to neutralize poisoned food and help ill with typhus. Europeans believed that lemons are excellent prevention of malaria, plague, scurvy and an antidote for snake bites. Also it was used to remove toxins, relieve pain in arthritis and heart disease.

Currently, the lemon is widely distributed in many subtropical countries of North America and Europe, in particular in the Caucasus, in Florida. Lemon essential oil is mainly produced in France and Italy. Lemon grown as a houseplant.

The composition and preparation of essential oil of lemon

Lemon essential oil is extracted from the rind of the fruit or fresh pericarp by cold pressing or distillation. To produce 1 kg of essential oil should be used about three thousand of lemons, in other words, close to 60-70 kg of raw material. Lemon essential oil containing limonene (90%), and terpenes, linalool, citral and other substances.

Properties of essential oil of lemon

Lemon essential oil is considered one of the *most popular and sold oil*. This status the oil deserved due to its unique healing and beneficial properties. It is very widely used in medicine, cosmetics, aromatherapy, cosmetics, cooking, etc. Industries.

Lemon and lemon oil are known primarily as an effective means for the *flu, respiratory and viral diseases*. It is especially important to use it in *hepatitis, herpes and other infections*. Because it has a pronounced antiviral activity.

The antibacterial properties of essential oil of lemon is shown *against tuberculosis bacilli, streptococci, staphylococci, and meningococcus.*

Coumarin, a part of lemon oil, *liquefies arterial blood, thus speeding up the process of circulation and promoting the regeneration of small blood vessels.*

Lemon essential oil - an indispensable way to cope with s*tress, improve mental and physical energy, as well as in the prevention of psychosomatic diseases.* Lemon essential oil is used to combat *worms, tapeworms and all intestinal parasites in general.*

Lemon oil has excellent *regulating effect on the liver, reducing blood flow to the liver, it acts as a general stimulant.* Equally effective remedy is lemon essential oil in vascular dystonia. It has a normalizing effect on the blood pressure, reduces blood cholesterol levels and prothrombin, prevents atherosclerosis, and therefore widely recommended in medicine for preventive and therapeutic targets for diseases of the cardiovascular system.

The action and the application of recipes essential oil of lemon

For therapeutic purposes, lemon essential oil is widely used in various fields. Depending on the disease it may be used in such form: inhalation, trituration, tubs and trays, internal use and spraying indoors.

1. Oil burner: insomnia, hypertension, fatigue and colds, as well as, if you want to neutralize smoke, light aroma lamp with 3-5 drops of essential oil of lemon.
2. Aroma bath: an excellent tool in the fight against rheumatism, cellulite, excess weight, get rid of toxins. For the bath, are enough 5-7 drops of essential lemon oil.
3. Massage: Use 5 drops of lemon essential oil for massage to help you with muscle pain after exercise, varicose veins and rheumatism.
4. Rinse: to remove bad breath or ease the pain in the throat with angina rinse your mouth with warm water and essential oil of lemon/1-2 drops in a glass.
5. Brushing teeth: daily cleaning of the teeth with the addition of 1 drop of lemon oil is effective in reducing gum bleeding, it prevents the development of caries and also qualitatively whitens teeth.
6. Compress: varicose veins, nosebleeds, apply a compress using 7-10 drops of essential oil of lemon on the emulsifier.
7. Inhalation: indispensable during colds. In 200 ml of water, add 2-3 drops of essential oils of lemon (duration of inhalation is not more than 5-7 minutes).
8. Internal use: lemon essential oil can be used internally for cholelithiasis, headache, atherosclerosis, hypertension, food poisoning, and to reduce the weight, take1 drop twice a day with tea, juice, sugar or a teaspoon of honey. Lemon oil - the perfect remedy against aerophagia: 5-10 drops of lemon oil is diluted with half or whole coffee spoon of honey in 1/2 cup warm water. Take 2-3 times a day.
9. Aromatization for liquid food: add 1-2 drops of essential oil of lemon in food, or in a glass of tea, juice.

Strong refreshing lemon flavor significantly *improves mood, inspires and refreshes.* Thanks to him, you will again feel the interest in the work and personal life. With its disinfectant properties, it is used for air deodorization.

The use of lemon essential oil in cosmetics

Currently, lemon essential oil is widely used as a unique cosmetic with antiseptic, detoxification, whitening effect - it perfectly softens, whitens and rejuvenates the skin. Lemon oil has the ability to *heal cracks in the skin, reducing brittle nails*. It can be used to care for oily hair - the lemon oil will make them shiny, helps get rid of dandruff. It is excellent as a massage oil for athletes.

Lemon essential oil for the skin

For *freckles, age spots and skin vascular pattern*, it is necessary to mix three drops of essential oils of lemon, chamomile 4 drops, 7 drops of wheat germ oil and 1/3 teaspoon of salt. The mixture is applied with a thin applicator on the field of pigmentation. Adding lemon essential oils in the cream will also improve the complexion, whiten skin.

In addition, the essential oil of lemon effectively fights against *wrinkles* – with lotion with the addition of essential lemon oil you need to wipe the face 2 times a week. *Brittle nails will be eliminated daily after application during the week.* In addition, it will give your nails shine and healthy form.

Lemon oil for hair

Dull, lifeless hair can easily and quickly revive with lemon oi, it will give them a luxurious natural sheen. To do this, after washing your hair, simply rinse hair with warm water with a few drops of essential oil of lemon. Especially elegant it looks, if you have light hair, because after this rinsing, they acquire a beautiful radiant hue. Oil of lemon softens hard water, and the hair becomes silky and obedient.

Lemon essential oil - one of the greatest gifts given to us by nature. The variety of its useful features and applications make it easy to achieve the desired effect even at home.

Rose essential oil: the use and composition. Useful properties of rose oil in medicine and cosmetology. Homemade recipes and treatment with essential oil of rose.

"Rose - the queen of flowers", is the name given to it, by ancient Greek poetess Sappho and still now the title remain unchallenged. From the ancient times, there are references about the rose and its magical properties in the annals of many states, and later rose even was declared a "paradise flower". Central Asian scholar and philosopher Avicenna wrote: "The rose oil increases the possibilities of the mind and increases the speed of thought." In medieval Europe rose was used for treatment of the oral cavity, the teeth, colds and headaches.

An interesting fact is that the more valued initially was the rose water, and the oil was just a byproduct.

Raw materials for essential oil rose

This natural rose essential oil is made only from the petals of a rose, or rather leaves from shrubs of the family Rosaceae. This is one of the most expensive essential oils. The high cost is due to the fact that it takes about 5000 kg of raw material to produce one kilogram of oil. In other words, to obtain a single drop of essential oils of rose, thirty roses are necessary.

The raw material for the production of the highest quality essential oil of rose growing on the territory of Bulgaria, just below the rank are Italy, Turkey and Iran.

Collection of roses flowers, as well as the choice of the place of its growth, requires a special approach. Just blooming flowers are picked by hand before sunrise, at the same time they do not get stale, and immediately sent for processing.

The composition of essential rose oil

Rose essential oil - a multi-component mixture, which consists of a solid part (stearopten) and liquid (eleopten) aromatic part. Depending on the method of distillation and habitats of raw materials, rose essential oil can vary in color from pale green to dark yellow. At low ambient temperatures rose oil becomes more dense in texture. It does not affect its beneficial properties, if the temperature rises again, it will acquire the properties of liquid form.

The use of essential oil of roses in medicine and cosmetology

Natural essential rose oil has a wide range of useful medicinal properties.

1. It has anti-inflammatory, antifungal and antiviral activity;
2. It focuses, improves memory, tones;
3. Calms overexcited when;
4. Normalizes the activity of the cardiovascular system;
5. Heals wounds and stops the blood;
6. It is an aphrodisiac;
7. Relieves depression, neurotic;
8. It helps to cope with insomnia;
9. Restores hormonal balance;
10. Eliminates bacteria overgrowth.

Rose essential oil is also called "*female*" oil, as it acts as an analgesic and normalizes the amount of *bleeding during menstruation days, eliminating the thrush, relieves postpartum stress.*

Rose essential oil is actively used in cosmetics for skin care and hair care. Acting on the skin, it *rejuvenates, smoothes fine lines, improves its firmness and elasticity.* In combination with other components, it *regulates the sebaceous glands, eliminates irritation and flaking, making the skin healthy and beautiful.* Moreover, it is used to remove scars and stretch marks.

Homemade recipes for the use of essential oil of rose

- To combat candidiasis at home: 3 drops of essential oil of rose (1 drop per teaspoon of soda) per 500 ml of boiled water.
- In occurrence of sudden toothache helps rinse solution at the rate of 1 drop of essential oil of rose (drop to a half teaspoon of soda) per 100 ml of water.
- Rose oil to improve the general well-being: is taken three times a day before meals - one drop of oil on a piece of sugar.
- Rose essential oil can be added to the bath (10 drops) *for stress relief, relaxation and improve skin and hair condition.* Due to the fact that the molecules of essential oils of rose rapidly penetrate the epidermis is not necessary to take a bath for more than ten minutes.
- You can also make a bath with a special blend that will make your skin soft and velvety. Ingredients: milk (1 liter), honey (1 tsp.), rose essential oil (10 drops). Milk with honey stir to heat, add the essential oils of rose and pour everything

into the bath. For greater simplicity and lower utility instead of milk-honey mixture are suitable glass of kefir or yogurt.

- Massage oil for lovers: rose essential oil (4 drops), sandalwood oil (5 drops), essential oil of ylang-ylang (1 drop), peach oil (50 ml).

Rose oil can "enrich" your cosmetics by adding 4 drops in the tonic, cream, shampoo, shower gel or hair mask, and you can make your own all-natural means.

The simplest thing you can do from the essential oil of rose - is *rose water*, which can wipe the skin instead lotion. This will require 250 ml of water and 2 drops of essential oils of rose. The regular use of this lotion *will eliminate the greasy skin-zone, will narrow pores, will remove "crow's feet" around the eyes*. Moisten two cotton in rose water and place the disc on the closed eyelids, it will remove the *swelling, and after several treatments you get rid of bags*.

- Mask-Scrub for the face and décolleté. Ingredients: Honey (1/2 tsp.), rose water (1 tsp.), ground almonds (2 tsp.). All mix, carefully apply to the skin, rinse with cool water after 15 minutes.
- Anti-Aging Night Cream. Composition: rose essential oil (3 drops), patchouli oil (3 drops), ylang-ylang oil (2 drops), neroli oil (2 drops), almond oil (30 ml). All mix, put into the refrigerator for two weeks, after 3 weeks you can use it. Apply on clean skin before bedtime.

Clove essential oil: composition, useful properties and applications. Essential oil of clove for hair and skin: recipes.

Clove tree - an evergreen tropical plant from family of myrtle, is the raw material for essential oil of clove. It reaches a height of twelve meters, and it grows in Indonesia, Brazil, on the islands off the east coast of Africa and Southeast Asia. And the oil is produced from the buds of the clove tree, and from its fruits.

The composition of the clove essential oil

For the production of clove essential oil you need unblown flower buds, first dried and then processed by water-steam distillation. In the production of oil from the fruits, they are collected in the period of ripening, in which case their aroma and spicy taste become identical with the buds one.

For one kilogram of essential oil of clove are required to eight kilos of buds or fifteen kilos of fruit allspice.

The main component of clove oil (85%) – eugenol- finds application in various fields - perfume and tobacco industry, pharmaceutical, dental, and even the development of means for combating insects. Feature of clove essential oil is also that it does not evaporate .

Useful properties and applications of clove essential oil
In medicine clove oil is effectively used for:

1. improve memory;
2. recuperation after disease;
3. wound healing;
4. treatment of vertigo;
5. treating respiratory diseases;
6. improve digestion, increase appetite;
7. prevention of arthritis, rheumatism;
8. prevention of influenza, SARS;
9. normalization of blood pressure;
10. reduce pain for sprains and accelerate the healing process.

To use the clove oil drip 2 drops of oil in a teaspoon of honey and dissolve the honey in half a glass of warm boiled water. Take no more than twice a day.

Clove essential oil is very useful for the female body, as it *normalizes the menstrual cycle, helps in the treatment of infertility, stimulates the generic activities, and also slows the aging process.*

For cosmetic purposes clove oil is effective at inflamed, prone to acne, skin. In domestic purposes clove essential oil acts as an *insect repellent*: mosquitoes, moths.

Essential oil of cloves for hair: recipes
It is believed that the clove oil helps to *speed up hair growth by expanding blood vessels and improving blood circulation.* At the same time it relaxes and relieves fatigue.

1. The easiest option mask, for stimulating hair growth: Mix 5 drops of clove oil and 30 ml of base oil. As a basic oil can act as an ordinary sunflower or olive oil, and almond, peach, coconut and grape seed oil or oil from germinated wheat seeds.
2. Mask for hair growth: Jojoba oil (30 ml), rosemary oil (5 drops), juniper (5 drops), essential oil of clove (5 drops).

The treatment must have the order of ten treatments with an interval of three days, pause, and for the prevention-do just once a week. Result - *shiny, obedient and strong hair.*

Clove essential oil for skin: recipes

Clove essential oil help to cope with *acne and oily skin problems.* With it can be enriched any neutral cream, and can be base for any mixture of vegetable oil .

1. Composition for oily skin: cream or oily base (10 ml), clove essential oil (2 drops), lemon (2 drops).
2. Composition for the treatment of acne: cream or oil-based (10 ml), clove essential oil (1 drop), geranium (2 drops), chamomile (1 drop).
3. To combat regular rashes: the base- oil from germinated wheat seeds (10 ml), clove oil (2 drops), lavender (3 drops). Apply the mask on your face, avoiding the area around the eyes, rinse with warm water after 15 minute.
4. For cleanse the skin from keratinized particles you can use gentle aroma piling of own cooking. Ingredients: oat flour (2 tsp.), water, grape seed oil (30 ml), the essential oil of cloves (1 drop), cinnamon oil (1 drop), oil of thyme (1 drop), lavender oil (1 drop). Alternatively, oat flour can be replaced by rice and a base oil and water or milk. On pre-cleaned and washed by water, aromatic skin, apply the mask, after five minutes strictly by the massage lines rub it with light movements. Then rinse with warm water.

Other recipes with essential oil of clove

Widely used for bath. The clove oil fit well with oils of mandarin, eucalyptus and myrrh in the proportions of 2 drops of each oil to a full bath, while the temperature of the water should be cool, and the oil pre-dissolved in a tablespoon of emulsifier (milk, honey, sea or table salt). The adoption of such a bath will *relieve from fatigue, both physical and mental, and help to cope with nervous exhaustion.*

Clove oil in particular, can be used in wet cleaning and disinfecting rooms to combat pathogens. To do this, at the rate of one liter of water you will need: clove oil (3 drops), eucalyptus oil (3 drops), tea tree oil (2 drops).

To get rid of *migraine or sudden headaches* can help massage of forehead and temple of the head with the following composition: clove oil (1 drop), chamomile oil (1 drop), lavender oil (3 drops), almond oil (1 teaspoon).

Eucalyptus essential oil: structure, properties and application of recipes. Eucalyptus essential for the skin, nails and hair oil.

The essential oil of eucalyptus - a transparent thin liquid, colorless or slightly tinged with a yellowish color. Eucalyptus oil have a distinctive, recognizable scent - resin-tart, is cooling and light.

Homeland of Eucalyptus - Australia and Tasmania. The natives called it an evergreen tree "diamond wood" and "the tree of life." Since ancient times, the beneficial properties of eucalyptus were used for the treatment of wounds and infectious diseases, to relieve muscle pain and fatigue, as a seasoning in cooking.

Now eucalyptus is common in many countries of the tropics and subtropics. For the production, eucalyptus tree are cultivated in Portugal, Spain, California.

The composition of the essential oil of eucalyptus. Production of eucalyptus oil

Eucalyptus essential oil obtained by hydro-distillation of the leaves and young shoots of fast-growing species of eucalyptus (spherical and ashy). From one ton of raw material is produced 5.3 kg of eucalyptus essential oil containing 60-80% of *cineol*. This high content of cineol defines the therapeutic effect of eucalyptus oil. Furthermore cineol, in eucalyptus oil are tannins, flavonoids, various organic acids and aldehydes, - about 40 components.

The properties of essential oil of eucalyptus

Eucalyptus and Eucalyptus essential oil has a pronounced phytoncide properties. It is widely used as an *analgesic, antiseptic, anti-parasitic*. Masculine scent of eucalyptus provides *fast recovery from stress and diseases, increases sexual energy and concentration, promotes disclosure of internal resources and intellectual capacity of the organism.*

The use of eucalyptus oil

Eucalyptus essential oil has been used successfully for spraying in the air. This not only *repels insects*, but also destroys a wide variety of infection present in the air. In addition, eucalyptus aroma have beneficial effect on the human psyche, relax atmosphere of conflict and promoting longevity.

Preparations based on essential oils of eucalyptus have a powerful *anti-inflammatory properties*, accelerate the healing of wounds and burns. In conjunction with undiluted essential oils of sage, yarrow, thyme, lemongrass, lemon balm, it neutralize the aggressive components of the latter. The ability of eucalyptus essential oil to remove accidental burns from other essential oils makes advisable its use in samples of unknown oils. It is used to *relieve headaches* and it is used as an *antipyretic remedy for fever*. Eucalyptus oil - *one of the most effective plant means that lower blood sugar*, which makes it useful in diabetes.

Use of eucalyptus oil

Eucalyptus essential oil - oil with dramatic effect. When applied to the skin it create sometimes a burning sensation, tingling, for 2-3 minutes, and a slight reddening. This is a natural reaction. But is possible and the idiosyncrasy of eucalyptus oil. **In addition, the use of essential oil of eucalyptus is not recommended for children under 2 years of age, during pregnancy for up to 4 months, and at the same time with homeopathic preparations.**

Treatment with essential oil of eucalyptus

For therapeutic purposes, eucalyptus essential oil is widely used in various fields. In various diseases use baths and inhalations with eucalyptus oil, massage and rubbing, internal use (after a doctor consulting), spraying the essential oil of eucalyptus in the room.

Recipes with essential oil of eucalyptus

During the epidemic of *influenza and acute respiratory infections* for the room air disinfection use spray with essential oil of eucalyptus. Use the oil burner or add a few drops of oil in a glass of hot water, put it on the battery or heater to speed up the process.

For *removal of muscular aches and pains in joints, rheumatism,* it is recommended massage and rubbing with essential oil of eucalyptus. For this purpose, a few drops of essential oil of eucalyptus is added to 50 ml of the base substrate (sunflower, peanut, soybean, sesame or almond oil).

Eucalyptus oil enriches the *blood with oxygen, thereby effectively improving respiration and nutrition of cells.*

In *colds and respiratory diseases, cough and runny nose* are recommended inhalation with essential oil of eucalyptus: 3-4 drops of oil, add 200 ml of hot water and inhale the steam for 5-10 minutes. *Using special inhaler increase the effectiveness of the procedure.*

For ease cold symptoms is effectively to take a bath with the addition of 5-7 drops of eucalyptus oil.

Use for mouth and throat rinse a solution of eucalyptus essential oil that *disinfects, reduces inflammation and pain in angina and other diseases of the throat.* Baths and compresses with eucalyptus oil are useful in *skin diseases, accelerate the healing of wounds, ulcers, burns and frostbite.*

Apply eucalyptus oil in gynecology for the treatment of *endometritis and inflammatory processes in the uterus and appendages.* In urology - *for cystitis and urethritis.* Effective action has eucalyptus in *prostatitis.*

As antibacterial option, essential oil of eucalyptus prevents the development of *thrush, herpes infection.*

Eucalyptus has detrimental effect on *staphylococci, wand dysentery and typhoid fever, paratyphoid A and B, inhibits the growth of purulent and anaerobic pathogens, dysentery amoeba and trichomonas.*

Spray in the air the eucalyptus oil, *is useful for emotional overload, it accelerates the recovery from illness and stress.*

The use of essential oil of eucalyptus in cosmetology

In cosmetology and dermatology it is widely used as for it *antiseptic, antibacterial, regenerating and deodorizing* properties. It is used for *skin whitening, treatment of boils and acne, to strengthen the hair and treat dandruff.*

Eucalyptus essential oils for the skin, hands, nails and hair

1. For oily skin, prone to inflammation, is efficient enrichment of cosmetics with essential oil of eucalyptus: 7-10 drops are added to 5 ml of the cream.
2. Skin wiping tonic enriched with eucalyptus oil, *effectively treats acne, promotes early recovery of the skin.*

Eucalyptus essential oil quickly relieves *irritation after insect bites.* It helps when it burns from contact with various plants.

Baths with the addition of essential oils of eucalyptus are effective *for prevention and treatment of fungal nail diseases.*

Addition of 5 drops of essential oil of eucalyptus in 10 ml of normal shampoo *strengthens the hair and effectively fights dandruff.* You can also rub a solution of eucalyptus oil into the scalp for 20-30 minutes before washing.

3. Eucalyptus oil can enrich hand cream: it *promotes healing of micro traumas and speedy regeneration of the epidermis tissue.*
4. Local application of essential oil of eucalyptus bleaches pigment spots on the skin.

Eucalyptus essential oil - a valuable gift of nature. The variety of its useful features and applications, make it easy to achieve the desired results at home.

Tea tree essential oil: composition and therapeutic properties Directions for use and treatment with essential tea tree oil.

From the outset, we must determine the order that the essential tea tree oil is not produced by processing tea leaves, this oil is produced by steam distillation of melaleuca tree components. Melaleuca alternifolia - so is called the tea tree, belonging to the family of myrtle, which grows in Malaysia and Australia. Tea tree can be both wild and cultural grown. Tea tree grows quite large, it is a long-living plant and well adapted to the climate fluctuations.

The composition of the essential oil of tea tree

Consists essential tea tree oil from 40% -50% monoterpenes, diterpenes to 40% and from 3% to 15% cineol. If the percentage of cineol is above, the oil can cause skin irritation. If diterpenes in oil are more than 30%, it indicates its high efficiency.

Medicinal properties of tea tree essential oil

Tea tree oil is considered to be particularly effective for therapeutic purposes, which is why in Australia, it is one of the essential components of virtually every medicine cabinet.

Being an excellent *antiseptic*, tea tree oil also has strong *anti-inflammatory and antiviral* properties. This explains its presence in the facilities for inhalation and massages for *colds, flu, bronchitis, sinusitis, cough and even angina*. Tea tree essential oil is also able to reduce the body temperature in feverish conditions. With a *wound-healing effect*, essential tea tree oil cures *burns and skin infections* (chickenpox, herpes, eczema), it neutralizes *poisons of insect bites*. Tea tree oil *strengthens the immune system*.

Tea tree oil – *is a great antiseptic*, it has this property, even to a greater extent than the known oils: eucalyptus and rosemary. Essential tea tree oil can affect both alone and combined with other oils. If the problems - are the flu, tonsillitis, otitis media, bronchitis or cough, it is recommended to do inhalations with essential oils of tea tree or use it in aroma lamps. To reduce the high temperature you should drink tea with tea tree oil: 3 drops of oil in a glass of warm liquid. Also during colds essential tea tree oil helps to stimulate the immune system of the human body.

The use of essential oil of tea tree

The spectrum of action of tea tree oil is wide, it is used for *acne and pustular infection*. It is indicated for *dermatitis -viral, bacterial and parasitic species*.

The oil is used in the treatment of *sprains, bruises, abrasions, cuts and burns*.

Another useful property of essential tea tree oil is that it perfectly complements the treatment of both *acute and chronic emotional disorders*. This oil is particularly indicated for people with *high anxiety and unstable mentality*. It is even recommended to always carry a bottle of tea tree essential oil in the event of urgent need to inhale the fragrance of the oil, to *calm the nerves*.

Not only to people prone to stress, but also to all others in difficult times, is recommended aroma of tea tree, it can be put on a scarf, neck, or even on a shirt collar. You will feel more confident, uninhibited and free, and to strengthen the effect of tea oil, it can be combining , for example, with *lavender essential oil.*

You can also improve *performance, concentration, relieve fatigue and improve body resistance, reducing the period of rehabilitation after diseases* with essential tea tree oil scent.

Even in the air, essential tea tree oil has a beneficial effect, its *disinfecting and preventing the spread of infection.*

Tea tree essential oil can be combined with other essential oils and can be used for cosmetic purposes in home conditions. The tea tree oil can be used daily for oily skin, it will help with the *itching, acne, hair loss, dandruff and warts*.

Methods of application of tea tree oil. Tea Tree Oil Treatment

- Trituration of the skin. In excessive sweating: mix and rub: 5 drops of tea tree essential oil, 2 drops of sage oil and 1 drop of essential oil of rosemary.
- Oil burner. In asthma attacks and bronchial asthma: 1 drop of tea tree essential oil, 1 drop of lemon balm oil, 1 drop of rose oil.
- Hair products. Shampoo may be enriched by adding, 5 to 10 drops of tea oil at once. You can also make hair conditioner and more useful. The same recipe can help those who are concerned about dandruff.
- If your hair is too dry, make a solution with 3 drops of essential tea tree oil and a hot cup of water and soak the combs in it and brush hair. You can spray same solution underwear.
- Lotion in the treatment of acne: 15 drops of tea tree oil, sage tincture 25ml., 60ml of "pink" water.
- Lotion for oily and porous skin: in 100 ml of warm (not hot) water, dissolve no more than 12 drops of tea tree oil and wipe clean skin.
- For herpes: make mixture from 5 drops of tea tree oil and 5 ml soybean oil.

Inhalation should be done as follows: in the freshly brewed tea, drip 3-5 drops of oil and cover with your hands, then exhale, open hands and inhale the resulting steam (repeat 5 times), then do 8-10 nasal breaths.

Bath: essential oil of tea tree 5 drops are mixed with 10 ml of milk (you can add honey) and pour in the water. The water temperature in the bath itself must be 37-38 degrees, and the bath - no more than 20 minutes.

Tea tree oil it is also used for deodorizing and for antiseptic baths for feet.

Before use, be sure to check the oil on the individual intolerance. Oil is contraindicated for pregnant women and children under the age of six.

Interestingly, help this essential oil can not only us, but our younger brothers, saving dogs and cats from the bad neighborhood - *from fleas.*

An important advantage of tea tree essential oil is that it has no side effects.

Essential oil of orange: the use, action and therapeutic properties. Essential oil of orange for skin and cellulite.

Externally, the essential oil of orange looks like a liquid fluid, of yellow-orange color, which has a sweet fruity aroma. *Essential oil of orange is today one of the most affordable and accessible essential oils.*

The essential oil is obtained from fresh orange peel by cold pressing and steam distillation from the peel.

In many countries, especially in America and Brazil, production of essential oils is combined with the production of orange juice. However, the orange essential oil obtained by this method is not very high quality.

The best in terms of quality is considered to be the oil from the Spanish and Guinean oranges.

Orange tree leaves are used to produce the Petitgrain oil, flowers – to obtain neroli oil.

You need to know that orange oil is subject to a very rapid oxidation. For this reason, it is usually added in it, antioxidant substances.

The essential oil can be obtained from both, the sweet and bitter orange fruits. The oil is contained in fruits, flowers and leaves, but its greatest amount falls on sweet orange peel. These two species differ in their composition and proportions of the active substances contained in the oil. Oil of bitter orange has a more delicate flavor.

The history of essential oil of orange

The homeland of orange trees is the East - China and India. In European countries, orange essential oil for medicinal purposes began to be used only at the end of the XVII century. In those days it was quite rare and expensive product. The first in Europe was used bitter orange oil. This juice of the fruit has been described by Avicenna in his, who used it as a medicine. In the XVI century Portuguese first began to import fruits and seedlings of orange trees from China.

Today, the orange trees are grown in many countries around the world: America (CA), the Mediterranean region, Mexico, India, Egypt.

The use of essential oil of orange

Orange essential oil has a fairly extensive application. Most often, it is used for the purpose *of skin care.*

Orange essential oil is suitable for all skin types. It *normalizes its fat content, makes the skin supple and smooth, helps in the fight against wrinkles, relieves muscle tension.* It also has *bleaching properties*, it helps *lighten age spots.* Displays toxins from the skin, softens the rough skin, so perfectly helps with *calluses.*

Orange oil for skin, cellulite

Orange essential oil has a positive effect *on dry skin, has a tonic effect.* Orange oil stimulates *the regeneration of dry skin, moisturizes and enhances blood circulation.* It is particularly indicated *for aging skin.* Great for oily skin, because it *cleanses and tightens pores* and helps *get rid of the scars* that left after acne. Orange essential oil also stimulates the *lymphatic system, reduces swelling and tumors.*

Orange essential oil is used to get rid of *cellulite.* Well it helps in dandruff, especially if you have dry hair.

Use the essential oil of orange and for oral care. Oil fights *inflammation and bleeding of the gums, cures disease, helps with periodontitis.*

Orange essential oil relieves *eczema, psoriasis and other forms of dermatitis.* It eliminates the *herpes on the lips.*

In the cosmetic industry the essential oil is part of lotions, creams, bath additives and deodorants. The aroma is the basis for perfumes and colognes.

The healing properties of essential oils of orange

Orange essential oil relieves *headaches, relieves muscle and joint pain, neuralgia, menstrual pain.*

Essential oil of orange *improves* the immune system. It is a good *antiseptic* that can be used for *colds, flu and infections of the upper respiratory tract.*

- Positively affect the essential oil of orange the gastrointestinal tract: normalizes the stomach, it helps to eliminate toxins, stimulates the appetite. It has a diuretic and choleretic properties. It is useful for preventing the formation of gallstones. It helps in cases of poisoning and constipation.
- Use the essential oil of orange for the prevention and treatment of diseases of the cardiovascular system. It increases blood circulation, normalizes blood pressure.

It promotes blood purification and reduce cholesterol levels. The oil is also useful in obesity and edemas.

Emotional effect of essential oil of orange

Essential oil of orange improves mood, can not only calm but also to tone up. Relieves fatigue. It helps to get rid of insomnia and feelings of anxiety.

Orange essential oil has beneficial effects on human bioenergetics. Orange oil helps to relax, relieves stress and depression. And it helps in the treatment of diseases which are caused by stress.

Essential oil of orange: precautions

Do not apply the essential oil of orange on the skin in the sun. This is because the oil is phototoxic – **accumulates sunlight and may cause burns.**

It is important to remember that in the owners of sensitive skin, long-term use in high doses may cause irritation and increase its sensitivity.

You should know that ingestion of orange essential oil can enhance the feeling of hunger.

Dosage of essential oil of orange

- For massage, take six - ten drops per 10 grams of base oil.
- For aroma lamps use 3-5 drops for five square meters of floor space.
- For full bath are enough 4 drops of essential orange oil.
- In the bath or sauna, you can add 3 drops to 10 g of water.
a) For application *to gums*, you should mix with other vegetable oil (1: 1). For regular oral care is recommended a drop of essential oil of orange in a glass of warm water, with it is necessary to rinse your mouth.
b) For enrichment of face masks, creams, tonics, shampoos are requires five drops per ten grams of base.
c) For inhalation: to 200 ml of water add two - three drops of essential oil to orange. Duration of treatment is 5-7 minutes.
d) For internal use you can add it to the juice or tea - one drop twice a day.

Orange essential oil may be added to necessity in the alcohol (liquor) and soft drinks..
Orange oil is widely used in industry, it is often used as a food additive.

Essential oil of Jojoba: the use, benefits and properties. Essential oil of Jojoba for skin and hair. Recipes with jojoba oil.

Natural substances have now become in demand as never before. Perhaps this happens because people are increasingly aware - *without nature help we simply die out*, and gradually turned into appendages of machines, as in science-fiction novels.

Natural materials and substances are in demand in all areas of life, we want to wear bio clothes, eat food grown in ecologically clean areas, live in houses made from natural materials and enjoy the same household items - such as furniture made from natural wood. Not surprisingly, the same trends in recent years appear brighter in cosmetology. A couple of decades ago, much less women wonder about the composition of cosmetics, but today cosmetic companies spend huge amounts of money to introduce into their production using 100% natural ingredients.

Natural ingredients are harder to obtain, and they are expensive. For example, spermaceti - a substance extracted from the cranial cavity of the whale, often is used in the manufacture of medical and other cosmetics. However destroying the whales was banned, and this can only be a happy moment - but what can now be added to cosmetics? *Artificial ingredients?* Fortunately, beauticians found a worthy replacement for spermaceti - jojoba oil, extracted from the seeds of the American shrub.

Jojoba oil - the arguments "for"

Jojoba oil is produced by a process of cold pressing, and it has a very rich composition - scientists say: *such chemical composition is no more in the world of plants.* Indeed, among the thousands of plants containing different oils, jojoba oil is the best - as demonstrated thorough and lengthy research. By the way, spermaceti, which mentioned above, also gives jojoba oil in its properties, so to exterminate whales is not need ...

Jojoba oil for skin care

For skin care use fresh and pure oil, obtained by compressing the seeds in cold conditions; *preservatives*!!! it does not need, that's why jojoba oil is hypoallergenic and can be successfully applied to any type of skin.

Composition of jojoba oil

The structure includes: amino acids and proteins, as well as vitamin E, which is so many that the oil differs by pronounced anti-inflammatory, antioxidant and regenerative properties. Jojoba oil can be stored for a long time and becomes bitter, and if it is added to other oils of vegetable origin, they also persist much longer. It seems incredible, but in the pyramids of ancient Egypt, archaeologists founded jojoba oil that retained it quality almost completely.

Jojoba oil has the consistency of a thick, but penetrates into the skin and hair, deeply and quickly without leaving greasy marks and creates a protective layer. Thanks to an excellent moisturizing and emollient properties, resistance to oxidation and temperature changes, jojoba oil is one of the best fat components used in modern cosmetics.

However chemists believe that - is a liquid wax, rather than oil. But for us it is important, because it is effective in *skin redness and inflammation, arthritis, acne, dermatitis, neurodermatitis, eczema, psoriasis.*

Jojoba Oil Properties

In the composition of cosmetic products, jojoba is perfect for skin care: *moisturizing and nourishing it deeply penetrates into the pores.* Most often, it is used as a base to which is added other essential oils, which when mixed with jojoba oil, will not lose its flavor, as it has no intrinsic odor.

The protective properties of jojoba oil are much higher than in other vegetable oils, so it's hard to find other oil than jojoba, *to care for the delicate skin of newborns.* The protective film formed on the child's skin, *gives the skin to breathe, but perfectly prevent waterlogging,* which can be caused by the use of diapers.

The action of jojoba oil

The skin of any type is getting better under the action of jojoba oil - particularly beneficial effect it has *on inflamed skin, over-dried and peeling skin.* Tired, fading and loose skin also needs this oil, it helps get rid of wrinkles. Jojoba oil treats *acne and minor injuries, relieves acne*; It makes *chapped lips soft and gentle*; It nourishes the *skin after shaving, sunbathing and swimming; softens scars*; It eliminates *stretch marks and fights cellulite.*

Jojoba oil for hair

For hair jojoba oil should be no less used than for the skin. Dry, brittle and dyed hair come alive after its application, as wax protects them, making strong and shiny. Jojoba oil should be applied to the skin in different ways. Clean oil can be applied to a small area of the skin, and on large areas is better to apply a 10% solution, which can be enhanced by adding other oils.

Jojoba oil at home. Recipes with jojoba oil

At home, you can add jojoba oil in *lotions, creams, shampoos and conditioners*, to do mixture for masks and massages.

- For example, it can be applied to the skin with a mixture of almond oil, jojoba or avocado: *daily after washing, shaving or sunburn. Wrinkles around the eyes* in the morning and evening can be lubricated with pure jojoba oil, adding to a 1-2 tablespoons of essential oil of jojoba, 1-2 drops of fennel or mint oils.
- A mixture of jojoba oil with essential oils of lavender and cloves or with cedar oil and kayaputa helps with many *skin problems*. Essential oils are added to the 1-2 tablespoons of jojoba oil – in proportion of 1-2 drops, 2 times a day mixture is applied on the problem areas.
- If you add to a tablespoon of jojoba few drops of oil of lemon balm, mint or rose, you get an excellent tool for *lip care*. Every day, in morning and evening, apply this mixture on your lips, massaging them easily, and they will become soft and attractive.
- *Cellulite and stretch marks* cause trouble for most women, And it does not depend on the age and body weight. In the first case it will help clean jojoba oil, although the addition of other essential oils did not hurt: lavender, patchouli, lemon, fennel, juniper and geranium, cypress or rosemary. The appearance of stretch marks can be prevented by using a mixture of jojoba oil, mandarin and lemon - 2 tablespoons of jojoba oil and 1-2 drops of oils indicated above. With this mixture you need to massage the problem areas or simply rub it into the skin.
- In *hair care* jojoba oil is not only added to shampoos and conditioners, but also rubbed into the scalp approximately 15-20 minutes. Dry and brittle hair will become softer and obedient, if several times a day you will comb them, with a few drops of jojoba oil.
- If your *hair falls*, then in jojoba oil add a few drops of oil of cedar, pine, eucalyptus, ginger and sage; With this mixture is also possible not only to lubricate the comb, but also make applications on the skin before head washing.
- *Hard feet skin, knees and elbows skin* become soft and well-groomed, if after a warm bath, you will rub in these areas jojoba oil. If the *skin on the soles is strongly callous*, make steam bath for feet, and after a pedicure rub the in skin jojoba oil, as much as possible, and its softening properties permanently eliminate this problem.

Today all kind of jojoba oil are increasingly used in cosmetics, and in many recipes it replaces triglycerides, mineral oil, squalene and lanolin, working much more effective and safer than these ingredients. We can only thank the nature for this wonderful gift that people have been using for more than 2000 years, keeping with its help: **youth, health and beauty.**

Essential oil of ylang-ylang: an aphrodisiac and use in cosmetology. Medicinal properties and application of essential oil from ylang-ylang.

In fact, ylang-ylang - is the name of the tree, whose flowers are used for the production of a unique essential oil. The name of these flowers in a literal translation sounds like "flower of flowers", sometimes also called the most aromatic oil.

The history of the use of ylang-ylang oil initially associated with cosmetic use. Fragrant wood, so is called ylang-ylang, which grows on the coast of the warm tropical seas, it flowers blooming purple, pink and yellow. From it yellow flowers is produced the most famous essential oil. Since ancient times women of southern coast, mixed oil of ylang-ylang, coconut and rubbed their hair. It was only at the turn of the XIX and XX centuries when were discovered the healing properties of oils of flowers from fragrant wood.

Essential oil of ylang-ylang - aphrodisiac

Today, aromatic essential oil ylang-ylang belongs to a class of aromatic adaptogens and is an *aphrodisiac*, it has an active influence on the increase in sexual desire. No wonder in Indonesia for a long time it is customary to strew the bed of newly married with petals of this wonderful tree. Today, oil is also widely used for the production of high-end perfumes.

Essential oil of ylang-ylang in cosmetology

In the cosmetic industry, essential oil of ylang-ylang is best known for its beneficial effect on the condition of *nails*, it can not only strengthen but also polish your nails. In cosmetics for skin, essential oil of ylang-ylang is added in order to prevent *premature aging of the skin, as well as to get rid of acne*. Essential oil of ylang-ylang in the deep layers of the skin acts by activating the growth of new cells and giving the skin elasticity, soft and velvety. With makeup with ylang-ylang are removed *irritation and redness of the skin*, oil is used to treat *dermatitis and eczema*, it also contributes to the restoration of thin and brittle hair, prone to loss.

Cure properties of essential oil of ylang-ylang

It not only has beneficial effects on the nervous system, restores strength and eliminating the irritability but enhances memory and helps to cope with depression. Essential oil of ylang-ylang is indicated in *encephalomyelitis, arthritis, rheumatism and gout*. It can help you *lower blood pressure, excessive muscle tone, normalize the menstrual cycle and relieve the problems of menopause*. Ylang-ylang is useful during *colds*, because it helps to get rid of a cough and runny nose. Essential oil from ylang-ylang is also effective in the treatment of *ulcers and infections in the oral cavity*. It is used for *loss of appetite and bloating*. Essential oil of ylang-ylang is able to regulate the activity of sebaceous glands and help in the fight against *boils, carbuncles and even scabies*. Inhalation aromas of essential oils from ylang-ylang helps to normalize the *breathing and heart rate*.

Essential oil of ylang-ylang and the human psyche

It is used to relieve *emotional tension and getting rid of feelings of fear, anger and anxiety*. Ylang-Ylang aroma gives *self-confidence, stimulate creativity, intuition and gives a feeling of serenity*.

Essential oil of ylang-ylang: impact on sexuality

But the greatest popularity is the ability of ylang-ylang to affect the sexual sphere of man, not for nothing, it is considered a truly sexual oil with a pronounced erotic effect, that increase greatly libido. **But, trying to evoke the feeling of love you should be aware of the possible individual intolerance to it flavor.**

It is also important to know that the essential oil ylang-ylang, with it intense flavor, may not only cause dizziness but also headache, so using it, especially in the early stages is necessary in small doses. People with low blood pressure, is better to completely abandon the use of essential oil of ylang-ylang due to its ability to lower blood pressure. Usually natural aromatic oils have no negative side effects, as well as not addictive effects. Only, it is important to make sure that the oil is really high quality and complies with international standards ISO, the quality and authenticity of the natural essential oils must be confirmed by the *USA certificates*.

Normally, a healthy person's skin reaction to the essential oils of ylang-ylang is neutral.

Although oil is indicated for children in night terrors, it is important to know that in the age smaller than 12 years is not recommended to use it, as well as oil of jasmine and carnation.

Terms of use of the essential oil from ylang-ylang

When you use the essential oil of ylang-ylang, important is to respect some rules:

1. You must be sure to check on the individual tolerance;
2. Use only high quality essential oil, as already mentioned; must comply with international standards;
3. Recommendations for the use of aromatic oils should be fully respected, it is necessary not only to strictly maintain the dosage, but also comply with all the prescribed precautions;
4. Only strict adherence to the conditions and terms of storage of essential oils can guarantee the safety and effectiveness of its use;
5. Do not deviate from the restrictions prescribed in the accompanying description and by your doctor, especially if you are pregnant women, children and people suffering from allergic diseases or prone to them.

Subject to the above rules, aromatherapy will give not only a distinct health benefits, but will also become way to deal with various problems and diseases. And if health problems do not bother you, then use the magical effect of the essential oil from ylang-ylang in the emotional sphere. Acting on the subconscious, the oil not only relieves the feeling of insecurity and anxiety, it loosens up, as if drawing positive energy and fills the world with love and harmony.

Ylang-ylang is considered magical fragrance and is meant for those who want not just to charm a loved one, and to ignite the fire of passion in it. It is also recommended to use this fragrance in oil burner to protect the atmosphere of the house from quarrels and conflicts.

The essential oil of rosemary. Properties, application, contraindications and treatment with essential oil of rosemary. Hair masks with rosemary.

Rosemary essential oil is made from a flowering shrub- Rosmarinus officinalis. The consistency of oil is fluid and light, have no color. The aroma of rosemary is fresh, but at the same time steady with bright herbal notes.

The properties of essential oil of rosemary

One of the expressed properties of rosemary essential oil is that it is perfectly stimulates precisely those brain cells that are responsible for memory. That is why the branch of a bush is considered a symbol of memories. The scent of rosemary in alternative medicine is used even when in amnesia. Earlier Greek students before exams done wreaths of rosemary branches and wore them during the exams to enhance memory, enhance concentration and improve mental alertness. The aroma of rosemary has always been loved by scientists, clerks and students, because it helps to remember not only the number but also the names and foreign words.

Rosemary belongs to the class of tonic and aphrodisiac scents.

The use and treatment with essential oil of rosemary

As a powerful stimulant of the immune activity of the human body, rosemary essential oil has a beneficial effect on the work of the digestive system, it is able to not only fight with inflammation, but also work as a choleretic agent.

Rosemary essential oil is used in case of problems with the respiratory tract, it and relieves coughing very fast.

The aroma of rosemary is considered the "heart of the fragrance." It regulates the function of the *circulatory system and the heart muscle, and normalizes blood pressure.* It have the ability to reduce the level of *"bad" cholesterol in the blood,* and have *anti-sclerotic effect.*

The aroma of rosemary is able to cope even with pain, acting as a *natural analgesic.* It is recommended to rub *the forehead, temples and neck to relieve a headache associated with a stressful situation.* This fragrance will be indispensable in the composition of funds for massages in aroma lamps or aromatic bath, if your goal is to *relax the body,* if you feel *muscle fatigue and lethargy.*

Fresh and invigorating it is also capable to restore the body's defenses and increase his endurance.

Even pregnant women can apply this oil, but only to get rid of nausea in the morning and using no more than 5 drops at once, you can also directly in this case, inhale the aroma from vial. Essential rosemary oil is an effective tool for the treatment of *vascular dystonia,* it can improve *cerebral blood circulation,* get rid of *eye fatigue* and even improve *visual acuity.* Rosemary displays from the state of fainting and dizziness while helping in those who suffer from hypotenssion.

On an emotional level, the essential oil of rosemary is able to save people from *insecurity, suspiciousness and excessive shyness.* The use of this oil is useful in post stress therapy as it quickly returns the *joy of life,* eliminating the psychological problems.

On the power of the person, rosemary essential oil also acts positively, helping to think clearly and encouraging to logical conclusions.

Rosemary essential oil will help, and after active exercise, he will definitely relieve pain of overworked muscles.

Rosemary essential oil in cosmetics

And, of course, aromatic rosemary oil is actively used in cosmetology. With it you may decrease the *increased secretion of oily skin*, it helps to reduce *enlarged pores*. Rosemary essential oil restores elasticity of the top layer of skin (epidermis) and softens the rougher areas. It is also used for the early disposal of scars, it is indicated in furunculosis and acne.

Rosemary essential oil has a pronounced anti-cellulite effect.

And if you want to quickly and accurately to sunbathe, take rosemary oil orally (1 drop of oil per cup of liquid).

Indications of rosemary essential oil

It is used for:

1. aromatic baths (5 drops per bath);
2. for making compresses, rubbing and massage;
3. with it saturate various cosmetic products (creams, lotions, shampoos, etc.);
4. may be taken orally;
5. fill with it aroma lamp.

Contraindications for the use of essential oil of rosemary

But even for this warm, spicy and very cozy aroma exists contraindications.

Mandatory verificate any essential oil on the individual intolerance. To do this, take a small amount of oil and apply it to the skin on the inside of the elbow and behind the ears (the sensation of arose burning should appear in a few minutes) and wait 12 hours if the discomfort does not arise, then the oil can be safely used.

Rosemary oil is not recommended for *epileptics, people prone to seizures and high blood pressure;* people with high blood pressure should be careful using this fragrance, although discomfort will pass no later than two weeks of use. In pregnancy is also better to except the oil. To avoid uneven tanning and sunburn, the oil can not be applied to the skin oil less than an hour before entering the open sun.

Rosemary essential oil for hair: mask with rosemary

Rosemary essential oil is also known for its beneficial effect on the hair and scalp. It not only removes *dandruff and stimulate hair growth*, but also to *stop hair loss and tones the scalp*, which becomes more healthy. For strengthen fatty or normal hair, use the following recipe hair mask with essential oil of rosemary.

- Take 10 ml of jojoba oil- base oil and 20 ml of grape seed oil. In the basis pour 2 drops of rosemary oil, 2 drops of calamus oil and 1 drop of birch oil and bay. Receipt of funds should be rubbed into the hair roots, after that cover head with a plastic cap and leave for 60 minutes, then rinse with warm water.
- To strengthen the dry and brittle hairs, take as base: 10 ml of the following oils- avocado, jojoba, macadamia. Then add 2 drops of rosemary oil, ylang-ylang, sweet and 1 drop of chamomile oil, birch and bay. Then proceed as in the previous recipe.
- If you prefer to mix essential oils with shampoo, then for women with dark hair suit the following recipe. Here for the basis is necessary to take 100 ml of shampoo for your hair type and add to it 6 drops of rosemary oil and 4 drops of lemon oil and wild carrot. All mix thoroughly and medicinal shampoo is ready.
- In order to strengthen weakened hair, make a mask with rosemary: mix with a little salt- 1 drop of rosemary oil, basil, black pepper, 2 drops of ylang-ylang and 2 egg yolks. This mask should be applied to the hair and wash off after 30 minutes. *If you do not want to apply the mask, just wash your hair with this mixture instead of shampoo.*

Try it, maybe spicy bitterness of rosemary - it is exactly what you need.

Patchouli essential oil. Production, use and properties of essential oil of patchouli. Patchouli essential oils for the face: masks, steam baths.

The plant itself named patchouli - is a perennial shrub native to the Philippines. Patchouli height not exceeding 90 cm, with long drooping down leaves and white lilac flowers. Patchouli - pretty whimsical plant and needs a fertile soil that drains quickly.

Preparation of essential oil of patchouli

Aromatic patchouli oil is obtained from young leaves of bushes, although they do not have no odor, the leaves a long-term pre-treated and dried with superheated steam. The consistency of the oil turns heavy and dense, of mustard green color, it can be difficult to remove from the bottle, it is recommended that the capacity where oil is kept to heat or warm in the hands or in warm water.

The main producers of this essential oil are India, Indonesia, Malaysia and China.

Plant name patchouli went from Hindi, and the first application of the oil was found in India, in which it has been used for medicinal purposes, and later it began to be used in perfumery. From immemorial times, patchouli oil was indispensable antidote for insect bites and even poisonous snakes.

The use of essential oil of patchouli

Back in Victorian times people used dry leaves from bush of patchouli, which were laid in the folds of the famous cashmere shawls to protect them from moths. In India, dry bags with patchouli today are a popular flavoring agent for laundry. Patchouli essential oil has long been used by perfumers to create fragrances of oriental type.

As a representative of a class of aromatic adaptogens, Patchouli is considered an aphrodisiac. Its flavor can be called a night aroma and inviting due tart warm and resinous notes.

Patchouli is considered to be the scent of creative personalities, because it stimulates the creativity in persons.

Properties of patchouli essential oil

Patchouli essential oil has a bracing effect on the human body, it coordinates the self-regulation processes and regulates the activity of the nervous system, and has a fairly strong antidepressant action. In alternative medicine patchouli essential oil is used as an antiviral agent, recommended in the flu, as well as herpes zoster and herpes simplex.

Applying essential oil of patchouli rectally, you can eliminate the inflammation of hemorrhoids. It is indicated for cystitis and urethritis, also has a slight diuretic and anti-edema effect.

Patchouli essential oil does not develop inflammation in the genital area. That is why patchouli oil is often a part of the funds for personal hygiene.

Patchouli essential oil, being a strong erotic stimulant, makes the libido stronger, and sexual relations more open and harmonious. Leveraging potency, patchouli promotes the renewal of relations, as well as rejuvenates the endocrine system of the body.

Actively working on the emotional, physical and mental condition of the person, patchouli oil helps to find a way out of any, even the most difficult situation that requires high concentration and attraction of intuition.

In the occultism is considered that patchouli oil becomes an obstacle for the development of vampirism-myth.

Methods of application of essential oil of patchouli

Properties of essential oil of patchouli: supply, smoothing, rejuvenating and refreshing the skin. It is especially suitable for dry skin prone to fading. Patchouli essential oil also soothes irritation and flaking skin problem.

Considered useful aromatic oil for hair, especially if it's dry, it also will help to strengthen nails. Patchouli essential oil will not only make your hair shiny and elastic, but also eliminate dandruff.

Helping to rapid healing of cracks in the skin, patchouli essential oil helps to complete the regeneration of tissues, gives stable effect in allergic dermatitis and eczema. Patchouli oil is actively used to achieve a lifting effect for firming the skin. It has a pronounced anti-cellulite effect.

Ways to use essential oils of patchouli are quite diverse. It is used for making aromatic baths, in different cosmetics (shampoos, creams, ointments, lotions), for massage, irrigation, micro-enemas, as well as internal use and flavoring for wine and tea (in dry form).

Before the start of the application is necessary to check the essential oil on individual tolerance.

Patchouli essential oil is contraindicated in pregnancy, gastritis and gastric ulcer (in this case, it only can be applied externally).

It is believed that it has complex flavor and you must approach very careful to it. Maybe you should start with the use of patchouli, as a means for the wardrobe and then the light and magical fragrance gently open its mysterious face. Besides, this neighborhood is not very liked by insects (moths and their larvae).

If you already love patchouli, be sure to try this oil in the following recipes.

Patchouli essential oils for the face: for mask, steam baths

1. Cream for dry and tired skin. As a basis we can take your usual cream. Take a 10 mg base in which add 2 drops of essential oils of ylang-ylang and patchouli,1 drop of grapefruit oil.

2. Mask for the face. For the basis you can take the avocado oil or almond to which add 2 drops of essential oils of patchouli and 4 drops of chamomile oil. Dosages are made on the 10 ml of base oil.

3. Steam baths for the face. In half a liter of water, add 1 drop of patchouli oil, and neroli.

4. Erotic flavors. For it manufacture you should take 10 drops of oil bases, odorless, to which must be added:

- 1 drop of patchouli oil, ylang-ylang, 2 drops of cedar oil and 3 drops of sandalwood oil;

- 3 drops of patchouli oil, ginger and bergamot, and cinnamon oil-2 drops;

- 1 drop of patchouli oil, 2 drops of essential oils of sandalwood and palmarosa, 3 drops of ylang-ylang.

You will have to plunge into the world of fairy-tale aroma of patchouli, where you will get a full sense of love, happiness and prosperity.

Thank you, because you found time to read this book. If you, after the reading of this book have some questions, you can find the answer to it, by sending me a letter to the email address: costeiandrei@yahoo.com

Can I Ask A Favour?

If you enjoyed this book, found it useful or otherwise, then I'd really appreciate it if you would post a short review on Amazon. I do read, all the reviews personally so that I can continually write what people are wanting.

42977437R00105

Made in the USA
Middletown, DE
26 April 2017